ロッタとハナの
楽しい基本看護英語

迫 和子
ジェーン ハーランド

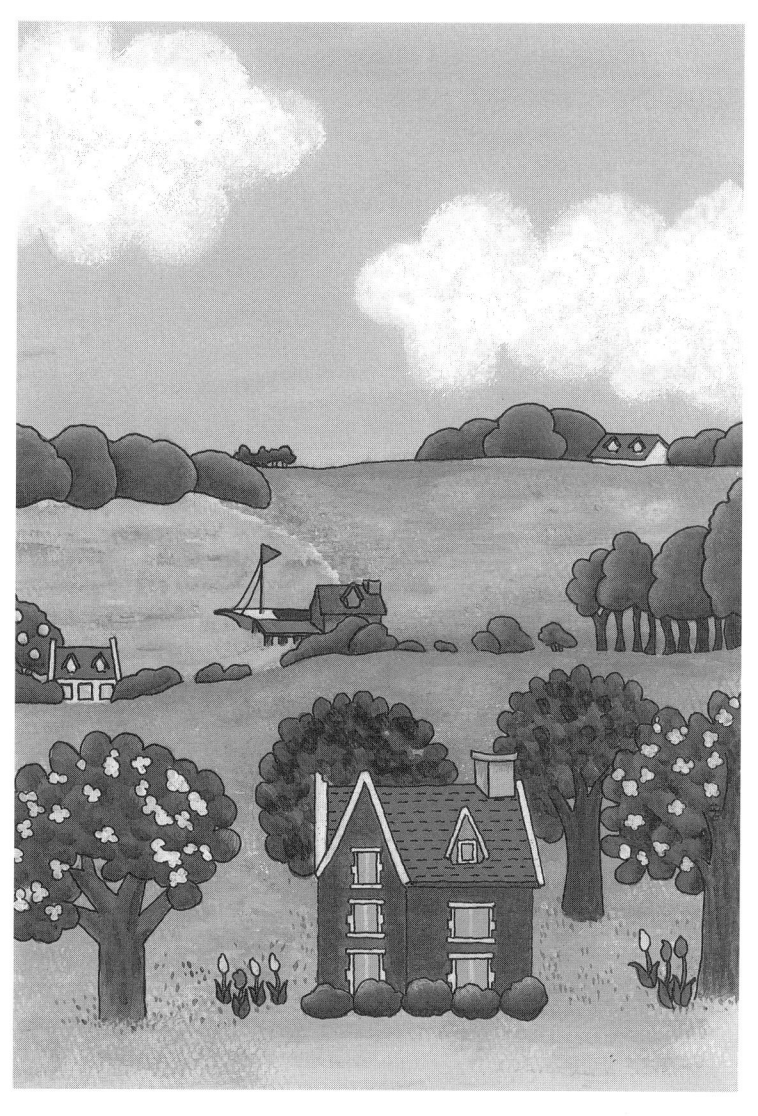

医学書院

● 著者紹介

迫　和子（Kazuko Sako）
西南学院大学大学院英文学専攻博士前期課程修了。国立南福岡病院附属高等看護学校，福岡女子短期大学，西南学院大学各校の非常勤講師を経て現在翻訳業。英国 The Economist 誌や医学・英語学関係の翻訳，英検，バイリンガル教育，英語教育法の研究に携わる。訳書──H.R. パッチ「異界──中世ヨーロッパの夢と幻想」（共訳，三省堂），同「中世文学における運命の女神」（共訳，三省堂）など。著書──「クリスティーンのレベルアップ看護英会話」（共著，医学書院）。同書は韓国と台湾でも翻訳出版されている。

ジェーン　ハーランド（Jane Harland）
英国国立シェフィールド大学大学院にて日本研究修士号を取得。福岡医療短期大学，福岡歯科大学，九州大学，九州大学大学院の非常勤講師，福岡大学人文学部外国語講師を経て，現在九州大学大学院国際教育センター・歯学府グローバル 30 にて講師を務めるなど，日本において 18 年間英語教育に従事。歯学英語教育，e ラーニングの研究，およびブレンデッドラーニング教材の開発に携わり，その成果を国内外の学会にて発表。Apple Distinguished Educators のメンバーとしてさまざまな活動を行う。

	ロッタとハナの楽しい基本看護英語
発　行	2011 年 11 月 15 日　第 1 版第 1 刷 ©
	2020 年 11 月 1 日　第 1 版第 5 刷
著　者	迫　和子，ジェーン　ハーランド
発行者	株式会社　医学書院
	代表取締役　金原　俊
	〒113-8719　東京都文京区本郷 1-28-23
	電話　03-3817-5600（社内案内）
印刷・製本	三美印刷

本書の複製権・翻訳権・上映権・譲渡権・貸与権・公衆送信権（送信可能化権を含む）は株式会社医学書院が保有します．

ISBN978-4-260-01410-6

本書を無断で複製する行為（複写，スキャン，デジタルデータ化など）は，「私的使用のための複製」など著作権法上の限られた例外を除き禁じられています．大学，病院，診療所，企業などにおいて，業務上使用する目的（診療，研究活動を含む）で上記の行為を行うことは，その使用範囲が内部的であっても，私的使用には該当せず，違法です．また私的使用に該当する場合であっても，代行業者等の第三者に依頼して上記の行為を行うことは違法となります．

JCOPY　〈出版者著作権管理機構　委託出版物〉
本書の無断複製は著作権法上での例外を除き禁じられています．複製される場合は，そのつど事前に，出版者著作権管理機構（電話 03-5244-5088，FAX 03-5244-5089，info@jcopy.or.jp）の許諾を得てください．

謝辞

　本当に多くの方々に支えられて，この1冊ができあがりました。
　David Gaal 氏，Mark Thompson 氏，Bill Pellowe 氏には本書の校閲にご協力いただきました．Thompson 氏と Kelly MacDonald 氏，Christie Provenzano 氏にはテキストの英語音声録音をお手伝いいただきました．
　ストックホルムの福祉センター元所長 Lotta Waernulf 氏，スウェーデン王立カロリンスカ医科大学の医師 Annelie Brauner 氏，Valdemar Grill 氏，Claes-Göran Östenson 氏，ストックホルム南総合病院の医師 Barbro & Finn Ouchterlony 夫妻，元看護学校ディレクター Monica Hellman 氏，ダンドリード病院看護師 Wiang Andersson 氏には，医療・福祉分野だけでなく北欧の生活全般についても多くの助言と情報をいただきました．Anders Olsson 氏，Erik Ollman 氏には，さまざまな海外リサーチを助けてもらいました．
　時政洋子さん，鈴木郁子さん，伏原美智子さん，九州大学芸術工学部工業設計学科の皆様には，それぞれのご専門分野でテキスト作成にアドバイスをいただきました．済生会福岡総合病院の皆様と藤本美奈子さん，西恵美子さんには医療・看護について，また，吉村松子さん，高瀬和子さんには看護英語教育について，共に貴重なご意見を頂戴しました．
　筆者の無理な要求に応えてかわいいイラストをたくさん描いてくれた桶谷房枝さん，MARIE さん．テキスト出版にご尽力いただいた医学書院の藤居尚子さん，吉冨俊平さんをはじめ編集・制作部の皆様．そして，いつもどこかで応援してくれていた，「クリスティーンのレベルアップ看護英会話」共著者の知念 Christine さん．
　本書の出版はひとえに皆様のご支援のおかげです．心より御礼申し上げます．

2011 年 11 月

　　　　　　　　　　　　　　　　　　　　　　　　　　　　迫　和子
　　　　　　　　　　　　　　　　　　　　　　　　　　　　ジェーン　ハーランド

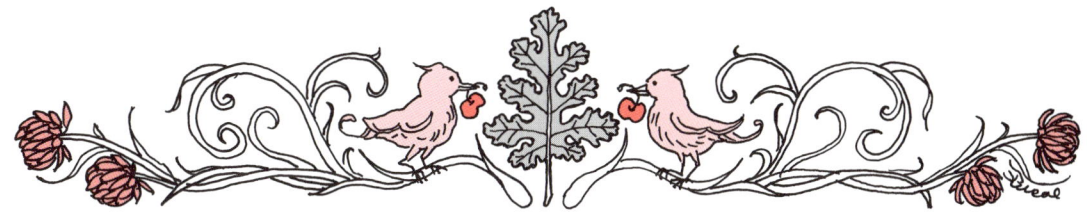

はじめに

　このテキストは，日本人の看護学生ハナが海外の医療や福祉に興味を持ち，スウェーデンに住むロッタにEメールを送るところから始まります。2人がそれぞれ自分の国の病院の外来・入院のシステムや看護の仕事，高齢者や障がい者の暮らしぶりなどを紹介し合います。

　本書のDialogやStep Up! Vocabularyのセクションは，病院内で役立つ英会話や基礎的な医療英単語など，看護英語の基本が学べるスタンダードな内容になっています。Storyの部分では，ロッタとハナの家族や友人をめぐる物語を楽しみながら，日本と海外の医療や福祉をテーマとする平易な英文を読む練習ができます。

　医療や福祉に携わる人が英語を学ぶのは，病院に来る外国人の患者やスタッフに対応するためでもありますが，最終的な目的はそれだけではないと思います。交通機関やインターネットの発達で世界の距離が縮まった今，より身近になった海外の情報を収集し活用することがますます重要になっています。そこで本書では，英会話と語彙の学習だけでなく，日本と海外の医療や福祉について書かれた英文を読むことも主眼の1つに加えました。

　筆者が縁あってスウェーデンに住み，生活者としてその医療や福祉を実際に体験した時，さまざまな点で日本とは考え方が大きく違うことに驚きの連続でした。本書が医療英語学習のお手伝いをすると同時に，みなさんがこれから日本の医療や福祉について考える新たな視点の1つとなればうれしく思います。

テキストの構成と使い方

- **Story**

　Storyは1つのテーマ（たとえば「外来病棟」）に関して，「ハナの章」と「ロッタの章」の2つのChapterで1組になっています。ハナの章にはタイトルに桜のマーク🌸が，ロッタの章には王冠のマーク👑がついています（王冠のマークはよくスウェーデンのシンボルのように使われます）。同じテーマについてハナの視点とロッタの視点を読み比べることで，日本と海外の医療・福祉の違いや共通点を見つけて楽しんでください。学習しやすいように1通のメールをAとBの2つのパートに分け，各200ワード程度にしました。Storyはテキストの後半になると，難易度が少し上がります。

- **Word List**

　Storyを読むうえでわかりにくい単語やフレーズを解説しています。Storyの第何段落に出てくる単語の解説か見つけやすいように，Storyの段落分けと同じようにWord Listも分かれています。

- **Dialog**

　各章のテーマに関連する，簡単な医療英会話を学びます。気後れせずに英語での会話に挑戦してもらうために，学生どうしのペアワークになっています。なるべくリラックスして，自然に言えるようになるまで何度も友達と練習してください。

- **Step Up! Vocabulary**

  医療英語の基本語彙を身につけるために，各 Chapter のテーマに沿った医療英単語のリストを掲載しています。覚えやすいように，対応する日本語訳はなるべく1つに絞りました。各 Chapter の Dialog とリンクしているので，この語彙リストを使って英会話の入れ替え練習ができます。

- **Exercises**

  各 Chapter で学習した内容の復習です。比較的簡単な問題を解くことで，自分がどれだけ内容を理解したかを無理なく確認します。

- **Puzzle & Game / Crossword Puzzle**

  Chapter が2つ終わるごとに，クロスワードパズルやワードサーチ，みんなで行うゲームなどがあります。Step Up! Vocabulary で学習した医療英語のボキャブラリーを定着させるために，楽しみながら反復練習してください。

- **Appendix**

  Step Up! Vocabulary の補足リストです。イラストはパズル形式になっているので，下線部を英語で埋めてイラストを完成させましょう。

- **Answers**

  巻末の解答ページはミシン目が入っているので簡単に切り離せます。必要に応じて事前に切り取り，保管しておいてください。

- **本書の記号の意味**

  （　）　①省略可能な語，②補足説明
  〔　〕　入れ替え可能な語　例：go up〔down〕stairs
  ［　］　略語　例：intravenous drip［IV］

英語音声の無料ダウンロードについて

本書をより効果的にご活用いただけるよう，本書の英語音声データ（Story, Dialog, Step Up! Vocabulary）を弊社ホームページにご用意いたしました。下記の URL にアクセスして，ユーザ名，パスワードを入力のうえご利用ください。

　http://www.igaku-shoin.co.jp/prd/01410/index.html
　ユーザ名　　lotta
　パスワード　hana

また，リスニング練習用ワークシートは下記 URL からダウンロードしてご利用ください。
　http://www.igaku-shoin.co.jp/prd/01410/ws.html

CONTENTS

Introduction

Chapter 1 Lotta & Hana ·· 6
    Dialog 1　　患者への自己紹介　7
    Dialog 2　　問診を始める　10
    Vocabulary　問診　11

The Outpatient Ward

Chapter 2 Visiting the Doctor ·· 12
    Dialog 3　　主訴　14
    Dialog 4　　その他の症状　17
    Vocabulary　症状　18
    Exercises　19

Chapter 3 Our Busy Hospitals ·· 20
    Dialog 5　　受診手続き　22
    Dialog 6　　外来　25
    Vocabulary　受診手続き / 外来病棟　26
    Exercises　27

    Word Search & Game　さまざまな症状 / 重症化ゲーム　28

The Inpatient Ward

Chapter 4 A New Family Member ·· 30
    Dialog 7　　入院準備　32
    Dialog 8　　入院病棟　35
    Vocabulary　入院準備品 / 入院病棟　36
    Exercises　37

Chapter 5 My Daughter's Arrival ··· 38
    Dialog 9　　検査　40
    Dialog 10　計測と数字　43
    Vocabulary　検査の種類 / 計測の用語　44
    Exercises　45

    Crossword Puzzle　病院案内　46

The Elderly

Chapter 6 Grandpa's Birthday ·· 48
    Dialog 11　診療科　50
    Vocabulary　診療科 / 院内の職業　51
    Exercises　54

| Chapter 7 | Grandma's House | 56 |

Dialog 12　日常の健康管理　58
Vocabulary　睡眠 / 食事 / 排泄　59
Exercises　62

Word Search & Game　院内の職業 / 道案内ゲーム　64

People with Disabilities

| Chapter 8 | Living Independently | 66 |

Dialog 13　日常生活動作　68
Vocabulary　日常生活動作 / 生活補助手段　69
Exercises　72

| Chapter 9 | Everyone is Different | 74 |

Dialog 14　病歴　76
Exercises　79
Vocabulary　病名　80

Crossword Puzzle　診療科　82

A Nurse's Job

| Chapter 10 | Hospital Training Begins | 84 |

Dialog 15　治療・処置　86
Vocabulary　治療・処置　87
Exercises　90

| Chapter 11 | Tough, but Rewarding | 92 |

Dialog 16　薬の服用　94
Vocabulary　薬の種類と服用法　95
Exercises　98

Epilogue

| Chapter 12 | In the Future | 100 |

Appendix-Vocabulary　体の部位 / 院内の備品　102
Glossary　107
Answers for Dialogs, Exercises and Puzzles　111

表紙・本文イラスト：桶谷房枝
本文イラスト：MARIE

Chapter 1 Introduction

Lotta & Hana

Story A

えーっと，何て書こうかなぁ…？

Dear Lotta,

I am writing to you through the introduction of your friend, Mats. He is an exchange student and I met him at the international festival in my town. He suggested that I write to you when I told him I am a nursing student and interested in foreign countries, especially their medical and social welfare systems. If you like, could we exchange e-mails and talk about each other's countries?

My name is Hanako Morita, but please call me Hana. I'm 19 years old and I'm studying to become a nurse. I often hear that Sweden has really advanced social welfare systems and I want to know more about them. I also like your country's pop music and fashion. Of course, I'd like to share a lot about Japan with you, too!

Best wishes,

Hana

Word List

*（ ）内は本文の行数

- exchange student（2） 交換留学生
- international festival（2） インターナショナル・フェスティバル
- nursing student（3） 看護学生
- medical and social welfare systems（4） 医療・社会福祉の制度

- share ~（10） （話を伝えて）いっしょに楽しむ，~の話を共有する

Dialog 1（患者への自己紹介）

Nurse: Hello, I'm Hanako Morita. I'll be your nurse.
Patient: Hello.
Nurse: Please feel free to ask me any questions.
Patient: Thank you.

Ⅰ．最初に覚えよう　　〜正確な会話のための〈必修フレーズ〉〜

1. Do you speak English?　　　　　☐ 英語を話しますか？
2. Could you speak more slowly?　　☐ もっとゆっくり話してもらえますか？
3. Excuse me? / Sorry? / Pardon?　　☐ すみません，何と言いましたか？
4. Could you say that again?　　　　☐ もう一度言ってもらえますか？
5. Did you say ~?　　　　　　　　　☐ ~と言ったのですか？
6. Do you mean ~?　　　　　　　　☐ ~という意味ですか？
7. What does ~ mean?　　　　　　☐ ~はどういう意味ですか？
8. Is everything clear?　　　　　　　☐ わかりましたか？

Chapter 1
Story B

Hello Hana,

Thank you for your e-mail. I heard about you from Mats. He is an old friend of mine and his family lives in my neighborhood.

Yes, I'd love to exchange e-mails with you. I am 26 years old and working at a school in Stockholm. The school has students aged 6 to 14. Children with and without disabilities enjoy learning together.

In my country, Japan is very well-known as a nation with advanced technology. Japanese food is also famous for being healthy, and there are many sushi restaurants in my city. I want to know more about Japan, a somewhat mysterious country for me. I'm sure I can learn many things from Japan. It'll be fun to introduce our countries to each other. Feel free to ask me any questions!

Best regards,

Lotta

Word List

old friend（1） 昔からの友人

I'd love to ～（3） ぜひ～したい
Stockholm（4） ストックホルム（スウェーデンの首都）
aged 6 to 14（4） 6歳から14歳までの
children with and without disabilities（4） 障がいのある子もない子も
learning（5） 学習，勉強

well-known（6） よく知られた，有名な
advanced technology（6） 先進技術
famous for being healthy（7） 健康にいいことで有名な
mysterious（9） 神秘的な
feel free to ～（10） 遠慮なく～する

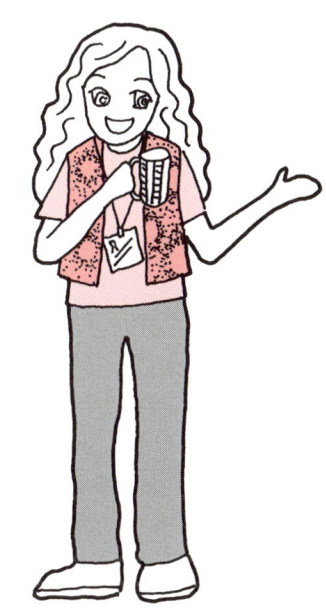

日本の話もたくさん聞かせてね

Chapter 1

Dialog 2 （問診を始める）

Nurse: May I have your full name, please?
Patient: I'm Carl Thomas Beck.
Nurse: May I ask you some questions?
Patient: Sure.

☆ 2人1組になり，自分の名前を使ってDialog 1と2を練習しましょう。交代して両方の役を行います。

Ⅱ．患者の基本情報を集めよう　〜問診〜

1. How old are you?　　　　　　□ 何歳ですか？【年齢】
2. What's your address?　　　　 □ 住所はどこですか？【住所】
3. Are you married?　　　　　　□ 結婚していますか？【家族】
4. How tall are you?　　　　　　□ 身長はどれくらいですか？【身長】
5. How much do you weigh?　 □ 体重はどれくらいですか？【体重】
6. Do you have any allergies?　□ 何かアレルギーがありますか？【アレルギー】
7. Do you smoke?　　　　　　　□ タバコは吸いますか？【喫煙】
8. Do you drink alcohol?　　　　□ お酒は飲みますか？【飲酒】

☆ 2人1組になり，英語で上の質問をしてみましょう。答えはもちろん架空の数字でOK！（^.^）交代して両方の役を行います。

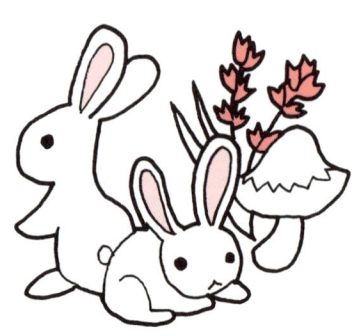

Step Up! Vocabulary

このコーナーでは，医療現場で使われる基本的な単語を Chapter ごとに特集します。難しい語もありますが，Exercises やパズルなどで繰り返し出てきますから，少しずつ慣れていきましょう。

問診　Medical History Taking

- ☐ family name   ☐ 姓
- ☐ first name   ☐ 名
- ☐ age   ☐ 年齢
- ☐ sex   ☐ 性別
- ☐ male / female   ☐ 男性 / 女性
- ☐ date of birth   ☐ 生年月日
- ☐ married / single   ☐ 既婚 / 未婚
- ☐ occupation   ☐ 職業
- ☐ address   ☐ 住所
- ☐ phone number (home / work)   ☐ 電話（自宅 / 勤務先）
- ☐ emergency contact   ☐ 緊急連絡先
- ☐ nationality   ☐ 国籍

- ☐ chief complaint   ☐ 主訴
- ☐ present medical history   ☐ 現病歴
- ☐ past medical history   ☐ 既往歴
- ☐ family history   ☐ 家族歴
- ☐ height   ☐ 身長
- ☐ (body) weight [BW]   ☐ 体重
- ☐ (body) temperature [BT]   ☐ 体温
- ☐ allergy   ☐ アレルギー
- ☐ drinking   ☐ 飲酒
- ☐ smoking   ☐ 喫煙

Chapter 2 The Outpatient Ward

Visiting the Doctor

Story A

Hi Hana,

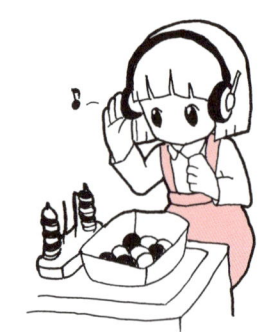

子ども用の聴力検査
ヘッドホンから音が聞こえたら
おはじきを１つ棒にはめる

Today, I will write about my daughter's experience so that you can learn about the medical system in Sweden.

One morning last summer, my three-year-old daughter, Karin, began crying hard because she had a bad earache. She often has ear problems, especially when she has a cold.

In Sweden, we do not usually go to a hospital unless the situation is quite serious. However, my husband, Erik, and I were worried about Karin's ears because she always has the same problem over and over again.

Erik called the local medical center, and the next day, he took Karin there to see our family doctor. Our general practitioner found a slight problem with Karin's hearing, and wrote a referral letter to an ENT specialist at a general hospital. Often there is a long waiting list to see a specialist, and you may have to wait up to one month!

Visiting the Doctor

Word List

▎ so that you can learn about ～（1）　～について知ることができるように

▎ earache（4）　耳の痛み

▎ over and over again（8）　何度も繰り返して

▎ local medical center（9）　地区の医療センター
　family doctor（10）　かかりつけ医，担当医
　general practitioner（10）　略語：GP＊　総合医，一般医
　hearing（11）　聴力
　referral letter（11）　紹介状
　ENT specialist（11）　耳鼻科専門医［ENT＝Ear, Nose and Throat］
　general hospital（11）　総合病院
　up to one month（13）　最長1か月

＊GP…地域住民のプライマリーケア（初期診療）を担当し，必要があれば専門医に紹介する。

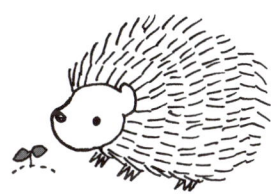

森で見かけた
はりねずみの赤ちゃん

Chapter 2

Dialog 3（主訴）

Nurse: What's the matter?
Patient: I have a bad headache.
Nurse: When did it start?
Patient: It started this morning.

☆ 2人1組になってDialogを練習しましょう。交代して両方の役を行います。
☆ P. 18のStep Up! Vocabularyを参考に下の会話を英語で行いましょう。
そのほかの単語にも入れ替えて練習しましょう。

1. A：どうしましたか？
   B：歯がひどく痛いのです。
   A：それはいつからですか？
   B：3日前からです。

2. A：どうしましたか？
   B：胸がひどく痛いのです。
   A：それはいつからですか？
   B：昨夜からです。

Story B

Three weeks later, I took Karin to the designated general hospital. Usually all patients pay a fixed fee before medical consultation regardless of their treatment. However, children under 18 years old, like Karin, can get free medical treatment in Stockholm.

Many hospitals in Sweden have a creative atmosphere with various paintings and small sculptures. Waiting rooms often have a play area for children even if it is not the pediatrics section. Karin enjoyed playing with a wooden slide and other colorful toys while she waited.

When we entered the consultation room, the ENT doctor stood up, shook our hands and said, "Nice to meet you, my name is Hans Olsson." He examined Karin's ears carefully. Then he explained in detail about the diagnosis, recommended treatment and what medicine she should take. The consultation took almost thirty minutes and the doctor answered all of our questions. This kind of "informed consent" is the basis of the Swedish medical system.

Karin was prescribed some medicine. We can pick it up at any pharmacy in town through the electronic prescription system. Her medicine was free because she was under 18. I am really glad that Karin's ears got better shortly after she started taking the medicine.

Lotta

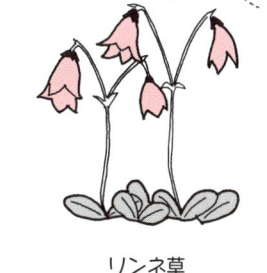

リンネ草
スウェーデンの生物学者
リンネの好きだった花

Chapter 2
Word List

- designated（1） 指定された
- fixed fee（2） 定額料金＊
- medical consultation（2） 診察
- regardless of their treatment（2） 治療の内容にかかわらず
- free（3） 無料の

- creative atmosphere（5） 芸術的な雰囲気
- sculpture（6） 彫刻
- pediatrics（7） 小児科

- consultation room（9） 診察室
- diagnosis（11） 診断
- recommended treatment（12） 推奨する治療法
- informed consent（14） インフォームドコンセント，説明と同意

- prescribe（15） 処方する
- pharmacy（15） 薬局
- electronic prescription system（16） 電子処方システム＊＊

＊定額料金…ストックホルムでは，総合医の診療費は 150 クローナ（約 1,800 円），専門医の診療費は 320 クローナ（約 3,800 円）（2011 年 11 月現在）。

＊＊電子処方システム…紙の処方せんではなく，各薬局のコンピュータで氏名や ID 番号によって薬がもらえる。

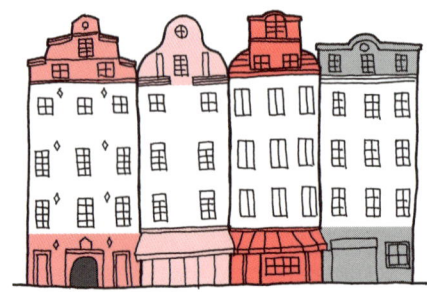

中世の古い建物が残る石畳の街

Visiting the Doctor

Dialog 4（その他の症状）

Nurse: Do you have any other symptoms?
Patient: I have a fever, too.
Nurse: OK, the doctor will see you shortly.

☆ 2人1組になってDialogを練習しましょう。交代して両方の役を行います。
☆ P. 18のStep Up! Vocabularyを参考に下の会話を英語で行いましょう。
そのほかの単語にも入れ替えて練習しましょう。

1. A：ほかに何か症状がありますか？
   B：咳も出ます。
   A：わかりました。もうすぐ先生が診察します。

2. A：ほかに何か症状がありますか？
   B：鼻水も出ます。
   A：わかりました。もうすぐ先生が診察します。

Reading Tips!

● 医療の一環としてのアート

文中でロッタは病院にたくさんの絵画や彫刻が飾られていることを話していますね。スウェーデンでは，アートは医療のツールとして役立つという"Art in Hospital"の考えに基づき，病院建築費の1％をアートに使う義務があります。このプロジェクトは1989年にUNESCOで始まりました。

スウェーデンでは「病院は最も美しく快適な空間でなければならない」という考えから，患者と家族がリラックスして過ごせるだけでなく，スタッフが快適で幸せに働ける環境作りをとても大切にしています。公立病院でも，看護師控え室や患者用の談話室など，インテリアの素敵な家庭的な空間になっているのを見かけます。この考え方は病院だけでなく，高齢者施設などでも取り入れられています。

Chapter 2

Step Up! Vocabulary

症状　Symptoms

- [ ] headache
- [ ] toothache
- [ ] earache
- [ ] stomachache, abdominal pain
- [ ] backache, back pain
- [ ] chest pain
- [ ] muscular pain
- [ ] joint pain
- [ ] sore throat

- [ ] 頭痛
- [ ] 歯痛
- [ ] 耳痛
- [ ] 胃痛，腹痛
- [ ] 背部痛，腰痛
- [ ] 胸痛
- [ ] 筋肉痛
- [ ] 関節痛
- [ ] 咽喉痛

- [ ] fever
- [ ] chill
- [ ] numbness
- [ ] cramp(s)*
- [ ] palpitation(s)
- [ ] dizziness
- [ ] nausea

- [ ] 熱
- [ ] 悪寒
- [ ] しびれ
- [ ] けいれん
- [ ] 動悸
- [ ] めまい
- [ ] 吐き気

- [ ] cough
- [ ] sputum
- [ ] sneeze
- [ ] runny nose
- [ ] hiccup(s)
- [ ] wheeze
- [ ] shortness of breath

- [ ] 咳
- [ ] 痰
- [ ] くしゃみ
- [ ] 鼻水
- [ ] しゃっくり
- [ ] 喘鳴(ぜんめい)
- [ ] 息切れ

- [ ] itch
- [ ] rash
- [ ] swelling
- [ ] lump

- [ ] かゆみ
- [ ] 発疹
- [ ] 腫れ
- [ ] しこり

＊通常，複数形で使われることが多い語には (s) をつけています。

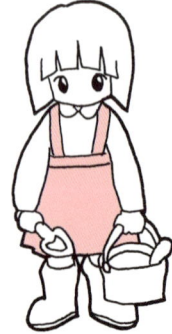

Exercises

Ⅰ．本文の内容について正しい答えを選びましょう。

1. Where did Karin have a pain?
   (a) her eyes　(b) her ears　(c) her nose　(d) her throat
2. How long did Karin wait to see the ENT doctor?
   (a) three hours　(b) three days　(c) three weeks　(d) one month
3. What did Karin pay for?
   (a) only the medical consultation
   (b) only the medicine
   (c) both the medical consultation and medicine
   (d) nothing

Ⅱ．次の文章を本文のストーリーの順番に並べ替えましょう。

1. Karin went to the general hospital.
2. Karin began crying because she had a strong pain in her ears.
3. The ENT doctor examined Karin's ears and explained about the diagnosis.
4. Karin received a referral letter from the general practitioner.
5. Karin's father telephoned the local medical center.
6. Karin went to the local medical center.

　　(　　)→(　　)→(　　)→(　　)→(　　)→(　　)

Ⅲ．該当する英語を右から選びましょう。

1. 熱　　　(　　)　(a) cough
2. くしゃみ(　　)　(b) sputum
3. 発疹　　(　　)　(c) wheeze
4. 喘鳴　　(　　)　(d) sneeze
5. 咳　　　(　　)　(e) runny nose
6. 痰　　　(　　)　(f) fever
7. 鼻水　　(　　)　(g) nausea
8. 吐き気　(　　)　(h) rash

Chapter 3 The Outpatient Ward

Our Busy Hospitals

Story A

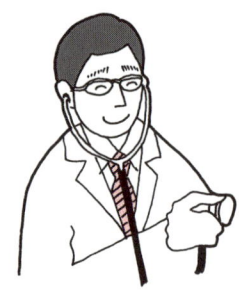

今日はどうしましたか？

Hi Lotta,

I was surprised to find out how different Swedish and Japanese hospitals are. In Japan, we have various medical facilities, from university hospitals and large general hospitals to small private outpatient clinics. Basically, you can choose any hospital and doctor, and visit on a convenient day. Appointments are not always necessary, especially when you go for the first time.

On your first visit, you need to fill out a patient registration form and medical questionnaire. You must submit these together with your health insurance card, and then you will be given a patient ID card. In Japan, everyone has to join the public health insurance system.

After your paperwork has been completed, you can go and sit in the waiting room. In Japan, people often say, "a three-hour wait for a three-minute treatment." It's common to wait a long time, especially at large, famous hospitals. Once I had to wait for over four hours to see a doctor!

Some doctors in larger hospitals see more than 50 patients a day, so usually they cannot spend a long time with each patient. It's difficult for the patients who are waiting, but the doctors and nurses are having a hard time, too.

Our Busy Hospitals

Word List

private（3）　個人の，民間の
outpatient clinic（3）　外来患者向け診療所
appointment（4）　予約

first visit（6）　初診
fill out（6）　記入する
patient registration form（6）　診療申込書
medical questionnaire（6）　問診票
health insurance card（7）　健康保険証
patient ID card（8）　診察券
public health insurance system（9）　公的健康保険制度

paperwork（10）　書類の作成，事務処理
a three-hour wait for a three-minute treatment（11）　3時間待ち3分診療

difficult（15）　大変な

Reading Tips!

● "I'd like to see a doctor" は「医者に会いたい」？

英語では "see a doctor" に「受診する」という意味があります。「風邪で医者に診てもらう」は，"see a doctor for a cold" となります。単に会いに行くのとはちょっと違うので，注意！

Chapter 3

Dialog 5 (受診手続き)

Patient: I'd like to see a doctor.
Receptionist: Do you have your health insurance card?
Patient: Yes, here it is.
Receptionist: Please put it in this box.

☆ 2人1組で Dialog を練習しましょう。交代して両方の役を行います。
☆ P. 26 の Step Up! Vocabulary を参考に下の会話を英語で行いましょう。
そのほかの単語にも入れ替えて練習しましょう。

1. A：医師の診察を受けたいのですが。
   B：予約カードはお持ちですか？
   A：はい，ここにあります。
   B：どうぞカウンターに置いてください。

2. A：医師の診察を受けたいのですが。
   B：診察券はお持ちですか？
   A：いいえ，初診です。
   B：どうぞこの書類に記入して（fill out this form）ください。

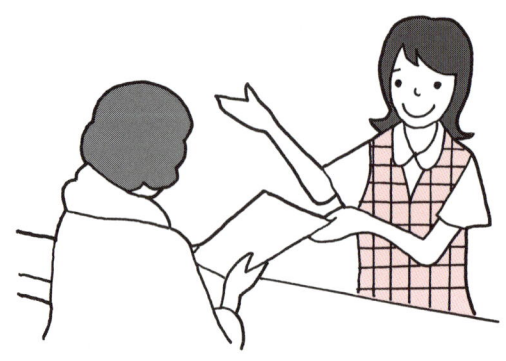

あちらの机でゆっくりご記入ください

Story B

After the consultation and medical tests are all finished, you pay at the cashier. On your first visit, there is a first consultation fee plus a medical test fee, a prescription fee, etc. You have to pay only 10–30% of the total cost as public health insurance covers the rest.

If you need some medication, you take your prescription to a pharmacy to get it. In the past, many hospitals had their own pharmacy, but now it's more common to buy medication from a pharmacy outside the hospital. Many people have a "medication record book," which is a small notebook to record all medications you have taken previously. It's really useful.

Under the current public health insurance system, the price is basically the same whether you see a famous doctor or a less experienced doctor. However, if you don't have a referral letter, you must pay extra at some hospitals.

Recently, hospitals and local clinics are working together. The clinics send seriously ill patients to hospitals, and also the hospitals ask the local clinics to treat patients whose conditions have improved. In this way, the hospitals and clinics cooperate to give the best medical care to the patients. Lotta, I hope you have a rough idea of the Japanese medical system now.

Hana

Chapter 3
Word List

medical test（1）　検査
first consultation fee（2）　初診料
prescription fee（3）　処方せん発行料，投薬料

medication（5）　投薬，薬
pharmacy outside the hospital（7）　院外薬局
medication record book（8）　お薬手帳

under the current public health insurance system（10）　現行の公的健康保険制度では
whether 〜 or ...（11）　〜であろうと…であろうと
less experienced（11）　経験の浅い
pay extra（12）　追加料金を払う

treat（15）　治療する
rough idea（17）　概略，おおまかなイメージ

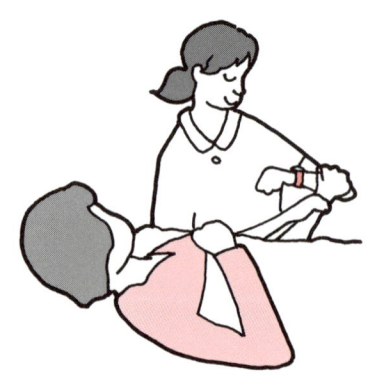

リラックスしてくださいね

Our Busy Hospitals

Dialog 6 (外来)

Nurse: Ms. Karin Anderson, please enter consultation room one.
Patient: Sure.
Nurse: Please sit down on this stool.
Patient: OK.

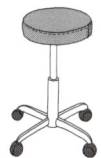

☆ 2人1組でDialogを練習しましょう。交代して両方の役を行います。
☆ P. 26のStep Up! Vocabularyを参考に下の会話を英語で行いましょう。
（下線部には相手の名前を入れます。）そのほかの単語にも入れ替えて練習しましょう。

1. A：＿＿＿＿＿さん，2番処置室にお入りください。
   B：はい。
   A：どうぞ袖をまくって（roll up your sleeve）ください。
   B：はい。

2. A：＿＿＿＿＿さん，CT検査室にお入りください。
   B：はい。
   A：どうぞベッドにあおむけに寝て（lie face up）ください。
   B：はい。

Chapter 3

Step Up! Vocabulary

受診手続き　Registration

☐	first visit	☐	初診
☐	return visit	☐	再診
☐	patient ID card	☐	診察券
☐	health insurance card	☐	健康保険証
☐	referral letter	☐	紹介状
☐	patient registration form	☐	診療申込書
☐	medical questionnaire	☐	問診票
☐	appointment card	☐	予約カード
☐	numbered ticket	☐	番号札
☐	medical chart	☐	カルテ
☐	medical certificate	☐	診断書
☐	prescription	☐	処方せん
☐	receipt	☐	領収書

外来病棟　Outpatient Ward

☐	outpatient ward	☐	外来病棟
☐	consultation〔examination〕room	☐	診察室
☐	treatment room	☐	処置室
☐	emergency room〔ER〕	☐	救急処置室
☐	X-ray room	☐	放射線室
☐	CT room	☐	CT 検査室
☐	MRI room	☐	MRI 検査室
☐	waiting room	☐	待合室
☐	general information	☐	総合案内
☐	reception	☐	受付
☐	cashier	☐	会計
☐	pharmacy	☐	薬局

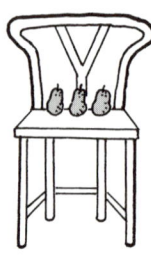

Exercises

Ⅰ. 本文の内容について正しい答えを選びましょう。

1. A "medication record book" is a notebook to write about...
   (a) your health check　(b) your medical fee
   (c) your medicine　(d) your hospital

2. Where do you go to get your medicine after a medical consultation?
   (a) pharmacy　(b) cashier　(c) reception　(d) nurses' station

3. How do the hospitals and local clinics work together?
   (a) The hospitals ask the local clinics to treat seriously ill patients.
   (b) The local clinics ask the hospitals to treat seriously ill patients.
   (c) The hospitals ask the local clinics to send doctors to treat patients.
   (d) The local clinics ask the hospitals to send doctors to treat patients.

Ⅱ. 初診の手続きを，本文で説明された順番に並べ替えましょう。

1. Go to the waiting room.
2. Submit the health insurance card.
3. Get a patient ID card.
4. Fill out a patient registration form and medical questionnaire.

(　)→(　)→(　)→(　)

Ⅲ. 該当する英語を右から選びましょう。

1. 健康保険証　(　)
2. 診察券　　(　)
3. 紹介状　　(　)
4. 問診表　　(　)
5. 処方せん　(　)
6. 診断書　　(　)

(a) medical certificate
(b) referral letter
(c) prescription
(d) health insurance card
(e) patient ID card
(f) medical questionnaire

Word Search 1　さまざまな症状

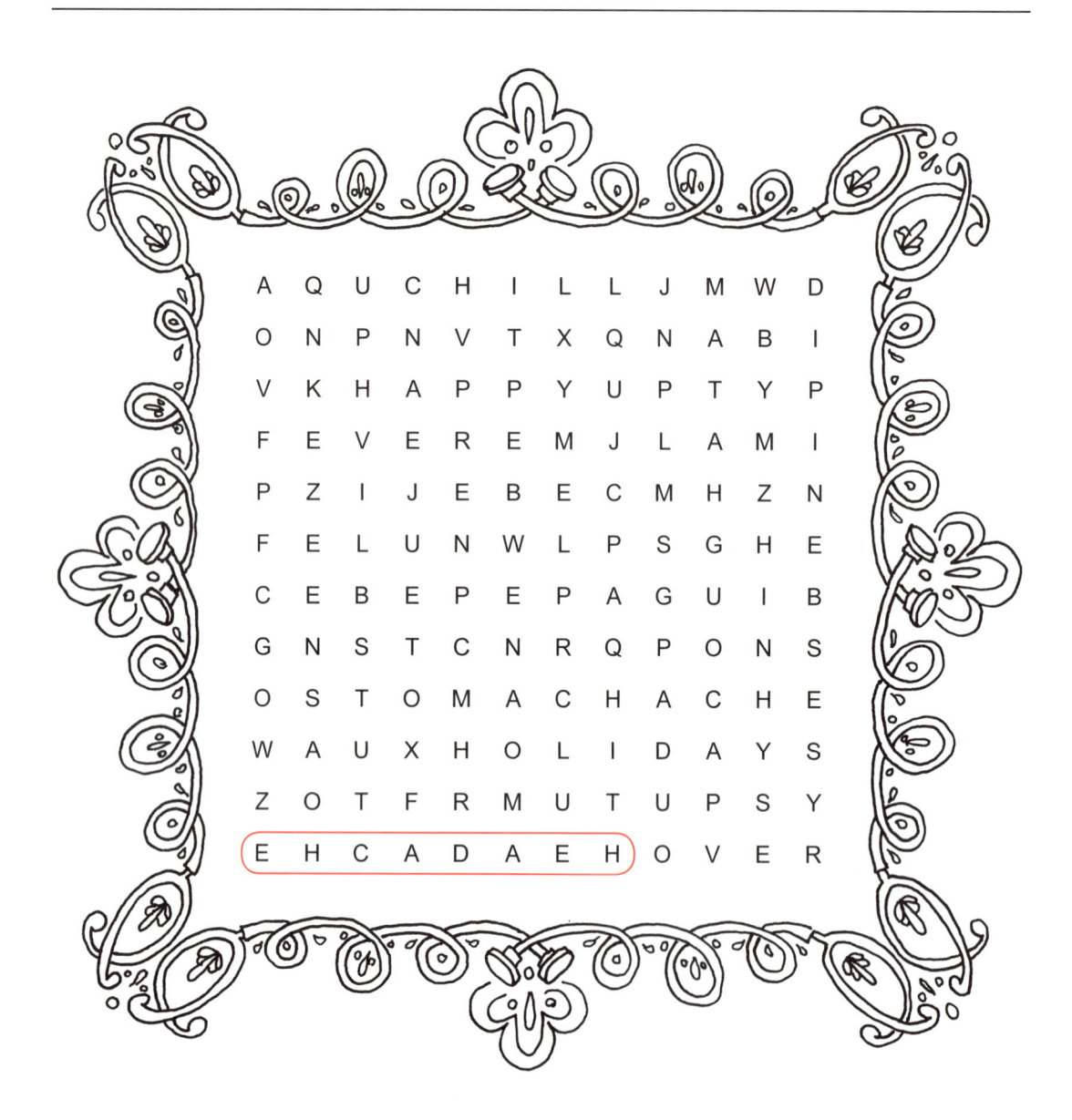

A	Q	U	C	H	I	L	L	J	M	W	D
O	N	P	N	V	T	X	Q	N	A	B	I
V	K	H	A	P	P	Y	U	P	T	Y	P
F	E	V	E	R	E	M	J	L	A	M	I
P	Z	I	J	E	B	E	C	M	H	Z	N
F	E	L	U	N	W	L	P	S	G	H	E
C	E	B	E	P	E	P	A	G	U	I	B
G	N	S	T	C	N	R	Q	P	O	N	S
O	S	T	O	M	A	C	H	A	C	H	E
W	A	U	X	H	O	L	I	D	A	Y	S
Z	O	T	F	R	M	U	T	U	P	S	Y
E	H	C	A	D	A	E	H	O	V	E	R

☆ 上の表の中に，さまざまな症状を表す英単語がタテ・ヨコ・ナナメに隠れています。探して丸で囲みましょう。また，各語を日本語で書きましょう。

1. headache　（　　　　）　　5. cough　（　　　　）
2. stomachache（　　　　）　　6. sneeze（　　　　）
3. fever　　（　　　　）　　7. sputum（　　　　）
4. chill　　（　　　　）　　8. rash　（　　　　）

Game 1　重症化ゲーム　"I have a fever"

☆　2〜4人程度のグループになり，順番に自分の症状を英語で説明します。

最初の人がたとえば"I have a fever"と言ったら，次の人は"I have a fever and a headache"と，症状を1つ付け加えて言います。次の人はもう1つ症状を付け加えて，"I have a fever, a headache and a runny nose"のように言います。4人目の人は，4個の症状を言うことになります。

症状が8個くらいになるまでゲームを続けます。はじめのうちはChapter 2（P. 18）のStep Up! Vocabulary を参考にしてもかまいません。

1回終わったら，順番を変えて最初からもう一度行います。

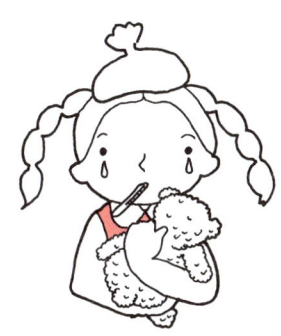

Chapter 4 The Inpatient Ward

A New Family Member

Story A

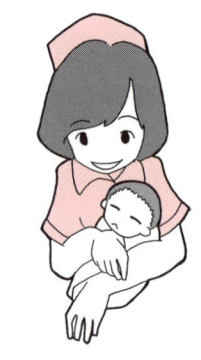

体重 3064 グラム・身長 50 センチ
とっても元気な男の子です！

Hi Lotta,

I've got some great news! My brother's wife, Mari, just had a baby! It's a lovely baby boy and they have decided to call him Ken, which means "healthy" in Japanese.

My brother was by her side at the birth and said he was really moved when the baby was born safely. In my parents' generation, it was very unusual for the husband to be present at delivery, but many husbands are these days.

The contractions started in the afternoon. At 11 p.m., the contractions were coming every 10 minutes, so Mari went to the hospital with my brother.

First, she went to a treatment room where a nurse checked her condition, the baby's condition and the progress of the contractions. Then she went to the labor room and had an NST.

My brother was by her side all the time and massaged her lower back. When the labor pains came, Mari used the breathing techniques she learned at mothers' classes. Recently, many classes are not just for mothers but also for fathers, so they are often called "parents' classes."

Word List

I've got some great news（1）　ビッグニュースです

by her side（4）　付き添っている
(be) moved（4）　感動する
(be) present at delivery（6）　出産に立ち会う
many husbands are (present) these days（6）　最近はたくさんの夫が立ち会う

contractions（7）　陣痛，（子宮の）収縮
every 10 minutes（8）　10分ごとに

treatment room（9）　処置室
progress（10）　経過，進行
labor room（11）　陣痛室
NST（Non-Stress Test）（11）　ノンストレステスト，胎児心拍モニター

lower back（12）　腰
labor pains（13）　陣痛
mothers' class（14）　母親学級

Reading Tips!

● 日本とスウェーデンの出産・育児事情

出生率……1人の女性が生涯に産む子どもの数を示す合計特殊出生率は，日本1.36人，スウェーデン1.70人（2019年）。

助産師……日本では男性は助産師になれない（2019年現在）が，スウェーデンでは男性が助産師として働いている。

育児休業…日本では子どもが1歳（場合により2歳）になるまで。スウェーデンでは子どもが8歳になるまでに両親あわせて最大480日（16か月）で，このうち最低90日は父親が取らなければならない。革ジャンに鎖をじゃらじゃらつけたヘビメタファッションの男性が，1人でベビーカーを押して子どもと過ごしている風景も珍しくない。ちなみに男女平等指数（ジェンダー・ギャップ指数）はスウェーデン世界4位，日本121位（2019年）。

Chapter 4

Dialog 7 (入院準備)

Patient: What should I bring when I enter the hospital?
Nurse: Please bring pajamas and underwear.
Patient: Can I rent hospital pajamas?
Nurse: Yes, but there is a rental charge.

☆ 2人1組になってDialogを練習しましょう。交代して両方の役を行います。
☆ P. 36のStep Up! Vocabularyを参考にして，下の会話を英語で行いましょう。
そのほかの単語にも入れ替えて練習しましょう。

1. A：入院の時は何を持ってくればいいですか？
   B：はしとコップを持ってきてください。
   A：コップは売店で買えますか？
   B：はい。

2. A：入院の時は何を持ってくればいいですか？
   B：スリッパとバスタオルを持ってきてください。
   A：バスタオルは借りられますか？
   B：いいえ，でも売店で買うことができます。

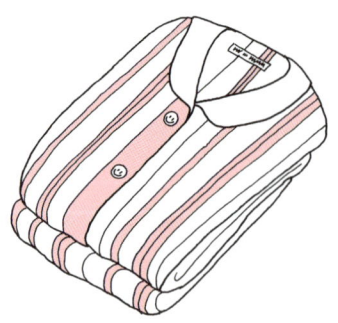

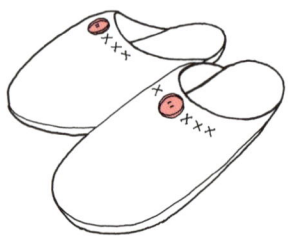

Story B

As the delivery approached, Mari went into the delivery room with my brother. A medical doctor, a midwife and a nurse worked together to help with her delivery. It was so painful that Mari wanted to get anesthesia but eventually she managed without it. In Japan, anesthesia at delivery is not always recommended as it could have negative effects on the baby.

Finally at dawn, the baby was born. He was 50 cm long and weighed 3,064 grams. This is almost the average size for Japanese newborns. My brother was allowed to cut the umbilical cord by himself. When Mari gave her baby breast milk for the first time, she couldn't stop crying because she was so touched.

Mari stayed in the recovery room for a while and then returned to her room. The baby stayed in the nursery for newborns the first night after the delivery. From the next day, the baby and the mother stayed together in the same room. Mari was in a four-person room, and it was filled with the energetic cries of four babies. It sounded as if they were taking turns crying.

If both mother and baby are healthy, they will be discharged after about a week. I'm really looking forward to welcoming the baby to our home. Please have a look at the attached picture. Do you think the baby looks like my brother?

Hana

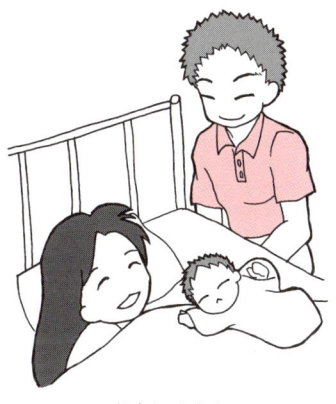

お疲れさま！

Chapter 4

Word List

- delivery room（1） 分娩室
- anesthesia（3） 麻酔
- manage without it（4） 使わずに済ます
- negative effect（5） 悪影響

- 50 cm long（6） 身長50センチ（特に赤ちゃんの身長を言う時の表現）
- newborn（7） 新生児
- umbilical cord（8） へその緒
- breast milk（9） 母乳
- (be) touched（9） 感動する

- nursery for newborns（12） 新生児室
- four-person room（14） 4人部屋
- energetic cry（14） 元気な泣き声
- take turns crying（15） 順番に泣く

- if both mother and baby are healthy（16） 母子ともに問題がなければ
- (be) discharged (from hospital)（16） 退院する
- attached picture（18） （Eメールの）添付写真
- look like ～（18） ～に似ている

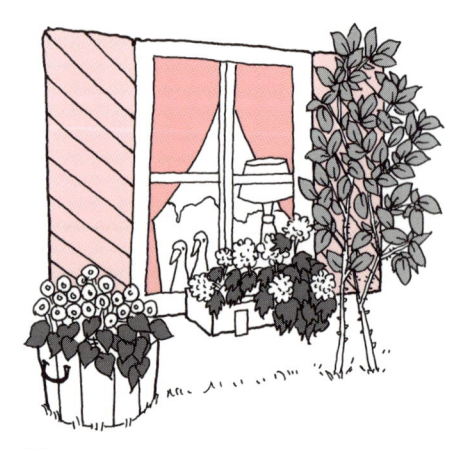

Dialog 8 (入院病棟)

Visitor: Excuse me, where is the nursery for newborns?
Nurse: It's next to the nurses' station.
Visitor: When is it open?
Nurse: It is open from 1 to 7 p.m.

☆ 2人1組になってDialogを練習しましょう。交代して両方の役を行います。
☆ P. 36のStep Up! Vocabularyを参考にして，下の会話を英語で行いましょう。
そのほかの単語にも入れ替えて練習しましょう。

1. A：すみません，食堂はどこですか？
   B：ロビーの向かい側（across from）です。
   A：いつ開いていますか？
   B：午前11時から午後8時までです。

2. A：すみません，シャワー室はどこですか？
   B：浴室の右側（to the right of）です。
   A：いつ開いていますか？
   B：午後2時から6時半までです。

Chapter 4

Step Up! Vocabulary

入院準備品　Preparation for Hospitalization

- ☐ pajama(s)　　　　　　　　　☐ パジャマ
- ☐ underwear　　　　　　　　　☐ 下着
- ☐ chopstick(s)　　　　　　　　☐ はし
- ☐ spoon　　　　　　　　　　　☐ スプーン
- ☐ cup　　　　　　　　　　　　☐ コップ
- ☐ towel　　　　　　　　　　　 ☐ タオル
- ☐ bath towel　　　　　　　　　☐ バスタオル
- ☐ tissue(s)　　　　　　　　　　☐ ティッシュペーパー
- ☐ toiletries　＜toiletry　　　　 ☐ 洗面用具
- ☐ toothbrush　　　　　　　　　☐ 歯ブラシ
- ☐ toothpaste　　　　　　　　　☐ 歯磨き粉
- ☐ soap　　　　　　　　　　　 ☐ せっけん
- ☐ slipper(s)　　　　　　　　　 ☐ スリッパ
- ☐ personal seal　　　　　　　　☐ 印鑑

入院病棟　Inpatient Ward

- ☐ inpatient ward　　　　　　　☐ 入院病棟
- ☐ nurses' station　　　　　　　☐ 看護師詰め所
- ☐ private room　　　　　　　　☐ 個室
- ☐ four-person room　　　　　　☐ 4人部屋
- ☐ labor room　　　　　　　　　☐ 陣痛室
- ☐ delivery room　　　　　　　☐ 分娩室
- ☐ operating room　　　　　　　☐ 手術室
- ☐ recovery room　　　　　　　☐ 回復室
- ☐ intensive care unit [ICU]　　 ☐ 集中治療室
- ☐ restroom　　　　　　　　　　☐ お手洗い
- ☐ bathroom　　　　　　　　　 ☐ 浴室，(婉曲的に) お手洗い
- ☐ shower room　　　　　　　　☐ シャワー室
- ☐ shampoo room　　　　　　　☐ 洗髪室
- ☐ laundry room　　　　　　　　☐ 洗濯室
- ☐ dining room / restaurant　　 ☐ 食堂 / レストラン
- ☐ lobby　　　　　　　　　　　☐ ロビー
- ☐ hospital shop　　　　　　　　☐ (病院の) 売店
- ☐ vending machine　　　　　　 ☐ 自動販売機
- ☐ emergency exit　　　　　　　☐ 非常口

Exercises

Ⅰ. 本文の内容と一致するものには○，そうでないものには×をつけましょう。

1. (　　) Mari went to the hospital when the contractions were coming every minute.
2. (　　) Mari got anesthesia because it was so painful.
3. (　　) A doctor, a midwife and a nurse worked together to cut the baby's umbilical cord.
4. (　　) Mari's baby was almost as big as the average size for Japanese newborns.
5. (　　) Mari's baby spent his first night in the nursery for newborns.

Ⅱ. 病院でマリが使った5つの部屋を，移動した順番に並べましょう。（実際には使わなかった部屋も選択肢にあります。）

1. delivery room　　2. labor room
3. recovery room　　4. operating room
5. four-person room　　6. treatment room

(　　)→(　　)→(　　)→(　　)→(　　)

Ⅲ. 本文の内容に合うように（　　）内の語順を入れ替えて英文を作りましょう。

1. 赤ちゃんが生まれたとき，彼はとても感動した。

(baby, born, when, moved, was, he, the, was, really).

2. マリは赤ちゃんに初めて母乳をあげた。

(first, time, gave, baby, milk, breast, her, Mari, for, the).

Ⅳ. 該当する英語を右から選びましょう。

1. 看護師詰め所　(　　)　　(a) inpatient ward
2. 集中治療室　　(　　)　　(b) vending machine
3. 洗濯室　　　　(　　)　　(c) emergency exit
4. 自動販売機　　(　　)　　(d) laundry room
5. 入院病棟　　　(　　)　　(e) nurses' station
6. 非常口　　　　(　　)　　(f) intensive care unit

Chapter 5 The Inpatient Ward

My Daughter's Arrival

Story A

Hi Hana,

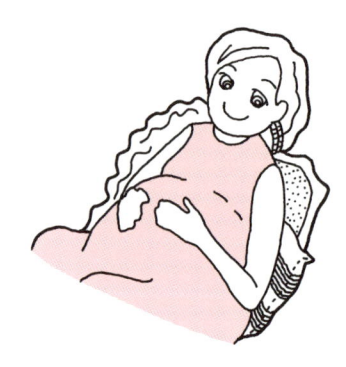

おなかの赤ちゃん
元気いっぱいですか？

Congratulations on your cute new nephew! Thanks for the lovely picture. Your brother's family looks very happy.

In Sweden, we go to a local maternity care center when pregnant, instead of going to a hospital. Usually we don't see a doctor if the pregnancy is going well. A midwife assigned to us gives regular consultations and support—checking uterine growth or the baby's heartbeat, giving blood tests and prescribing iron pills in the case of anemia, etc.

There are no medical fees for regular pregnancy checkups or for delivery in Sweden. We can have the midwife's consultation once a month after 20 weeks of our first pregnancy, or after 25 weeks if we have had children before.

Between 16–20 weeks of pregnancy, we go to our regional general hospital and have ultrasound tests. At this time, I got a DVD of a moving image of the baby inside me!

During the later stages of pregnancy, both parents attend classes about the birth and care of their baby. I hear that more than 90% of partners are present during the child's birth in Sweden. Partners can be present even if it is a Caesarian section, and not a natural birth.

Word List

congratulations on ～（1）　～おめでとう

maternity care center（3）　妊産婦保健センター
pregnant（3）　妊娠している
assigned to ～（5）　～を担当する
uterine growth（6）　子宮の発育
baby's heartbeat（6）　胎児の心音
blood test（6）　血液検査
iron pill（7）　鉄剤
anemia（7）　貧血

there are no medical fees for ～（8）　～には医療費がかからない
pregnancy checkup（8）　妊婦健診
after 20 weeks of our first pregnancy（9）　初めての妊娠の場合は第20週以降
if we have had children before（10）　前に出産経験がある場合は

ultrasound test（12）　超音波検査
moving image（12）　動画
inside me（13）　私のおなかの中の

during the later stages of pregnancy（14）　妊娠後半になると
partner（15）　パートナー＊
Caesarean section（17）　帝王切開
natural birth（17）　自然分娩

＊パートナー…スウェーデンでは90％以上のカップルが同棲期間を経て結婚すると言われているので，必ずしも赤ちゃんの父親が「夫」という立場であるとは限らない。

Chapter 5

Dialog 9（検査）

Nurse: You are going to have an abdominal echogram today.
Patient: What kind of test is that?
Nurse: It's to check your baby's condition using ultrasound.

☆ 2人1組になってDialogを練習しましょう。交代して両方の役を行います。
☆ P. 44のStep Up! Vocabularyを参考にして，下の会話を英語で行いましょう。
そのほかの単語にも入れ替えて練習しましょう。

1. A：今日は脳のMRI検査（brain MRI）があります。
   B：どんな検査ですか？
   A：電磁波（magnetic waves）を使って脳を調べます。

2. A：今日は心電図検査があります。
   B：どんな検査ですか？
   A：弱い電気信号（weak electric signals）を使って心臓を調べます。

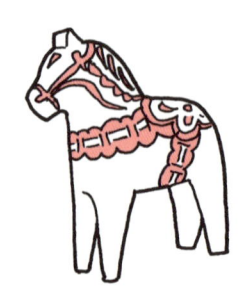

北欧の木彫りの馬は
昔の子どものあそび道具

My Daughter's Arrival

Story B

When you are hospitalized to have a baby, your partner's bed and meals will also be prepared upon your request. If there is no problem during the delivery, a midwife and a nurse will be in charge without a doctor. If you need anesthesia when giving birth, you can choose from various kinds.

I'll never forget the moment when Karin was born. In Sweden, we think it is very important for the family to be alone for a while after the baby is born. The medical staff left us alone immediately when they finished the treatments after childbirth. Our naked baby was on my belly. My husband and I enjoyed a peaceful time with the baby for more than one hour.

Karin weighed 3,720 grams. This was heavier than 3,400 grams, the average weight for Swedish newborns. I think Swedish babies are generally bigger than Japanese babies. Adults in Sweden are generally larger than Japanese adults with an average height of over 180 cm for men and 167 cm for women.

You can register your baby's name with the government anytime within three months, so some babies are nameless for a while. You can usually leave the hospital one or two days after the delivery. Then, it's time to start life with your new baby!

Lotta

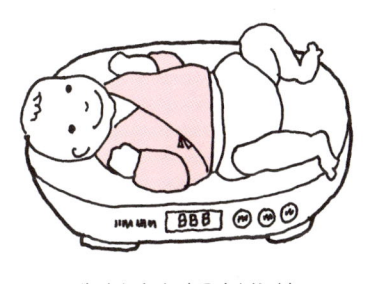

生まれたときのカリンは
やや太め

Chapter 5

Word List

- (be) hospitalized（1） 入院する
- upon your request（2） 希望すれば＊
- in charge（3） 担当する
- various kinds（4） いろいろな種類

- on my belly（8） おなかの上に乗せて
- peaceful（9） 至福の，穏やかな

- average weight（10） 平均体重
- generally（11） 一般的に
- average height（13） 平均身長

- register ～ with …（14） ～を…に登録する
- nameless（15） 名前がない

＊病室に家族の宿泊を希望する場合は，ベッド・朝食付きで1泊250クローナ（約3,000円）程度（2011年11月現在）。

Speaking Tips!

● 数字の読み方

- ☐ 167 cm　　one hundred (and) sixty-seven centimeters
- ☐ 3,720 g　　three thousand seven hundred twenty grams
- ☐ 36.8℃　　thirty-six point eight degrees (Celsius / centigrade)
- ☐ 98.6℉　　ninety-eight point six degrees (Fahrenheit)
- ☐ 上が154，下が95（血圧）　　one fifty-four over ninety-five

My Daughter's Arrival

Dialog 10 (計測と数字)

Nurse: How high is your temperature now?
Patient: It's 36.8℃.
Nurse: It went down a little.

☆ 2人1組になってDialogを練習しましょう。交代して両方の役を行います。
☆ P. 44のStep Up! Vocabularyを参考にして，下の会話を英語で行いましょう。
そのほかの単語にも入れ替えて練習しましょう。

1. A：（あなたの）血圧は今どれくらいですか（how high）？
   B：上が150，下が90です。
   A：少し高いですね。

2. A：（あなたの）お子さんの身長は今どれくらいですか（how tall）？
   B：90センチです。
   A：とても大きくなりましたね（really big）！

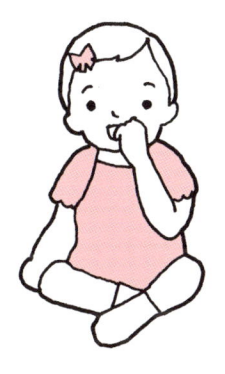

ちょっぴり女の子らしくなりました

Chapter 5

Step Up! Vocabulary

検査の種類　Medical Tests

- [ ] ultrasound, echogram, echography
- [ ] computerized tomography [CT scan]
- [ ] magnetic resonance imaging [MRI]
- [ ] electrocardiogram [ECG, EKG]
- [ ] electroencephalogram [EEG]
- [ ] X-ray
- [ ] gastroscopy
- [ ] colonoscopy
- [ ] urine test
- [ ] stool test
- [ ] blood test
- [ ] vision test
- [ ] hearing test

- [ ] 超音波検査，エコー検査
- [ ] CT 検査，コンピュータ断層撮影
- [ ] MRI 検査，磁気共鳴断層撮影
- [ ] 心電図検査
- [ ] 脳波検査
- [ ] X 線，レントゲン
- [ ] 胃（内視）鏡検査
- [ ] 大腸（内視）鏡検査
- [ ] 尿検査
- [ ] 検便
- [ ] 血液検査
- [ ] 視力検査
- [ ] 聴力検査

計測の用語　Measurements

- [ ] height*
- [ ] (body) weight [BW]*
- [ ] (body) temperature [BT]*
- [ ] blood pressure [BP]
- [ ] respiration
- [ ] pulse
- [ ] heart rate [HR]
- [ ] vital signs [VS]

- [ ] abdominal circumference [AC]
- [ ] body mass index [BMI]

- [ ] high / low
- [ ] rapid / slow
- [ ] go up / go down
- [ ] increase / decrease

- [ ] 身長
- [ ] 体重
- [ ] 体温
- [ ] 血圧
- [ ] 呼吸
- [ ] 脈拍
- [ ] 心拍数
- [ ] バイタルサイン（体温，血圧，呼吸数，脈拍または心拍数など）

- [ ] 腹囲
- [ ] 肥満度指数，体格指数

- [ ] 高い / 低い（体温，血圧など）
- [ ] 速い / 遅い（脈拍，呼吸など）
- [ ] 上昇する / 下降する（体温，血圧など）
- [ ] 増加する / 減少する（体重など）

＊Chapter 1 既出

My Daughter's Arrival

Exercises

Ⅰ. 本文の内容と一致するものには○，そうでないものには×をつけましょう。
1. (　　) There are no medical fees for regular pregnancy checkups in Sweden.
2. (　　) Pregnant women can have ultrasound tests at local maternity care centers.
3. (　　) People can have midwife's consultations twice a month after 20 weeks of pregnancy.
4. (　　) Partners of pregnant women can be present even at Caesarian sections.
5. (　　) Lotta's baby was taken to the newborn nursery soon after birth.
6. (　　) A baby's name must be registered with the government within three weeks.

Ⅱ. 次の数字を英語で言いましょう。
1. 158 cm（身長）
2. 46.3 kg（体重）
3. 37.5℃（体温）
4. 上が135，下が82（血圧）

Ⅲ. 該当する検査名を右から選びましょう。
1. EEG　　　　　(　　)　　(a) 胃内視鏡検査
2. ECG　　　　　(　　)　　(b) 大腸内視鏡検査
3. CT scan　　　 (　　)　　(c) 脳波検査
4. colonoscopy　 (　　)　　(d) 超音波検査
5. echogram　　 (　　)　　(e) 心電図検査
6. gastroscopy　 (　　)　　(f) コンピュータ断層撮影

Crossword Puzzle 1　病院案内

☆　下の空欄には病院内のいろいろな場所の名前が入ります。ヒントの英文と [　　] 内の選択肢を参考にして，空欄を英語で埋めましょう。難しい場合は Chapter 3（P. 26）と Chapter 4（P. 36）の Step Up! Vocabulary を参考にしましょう。

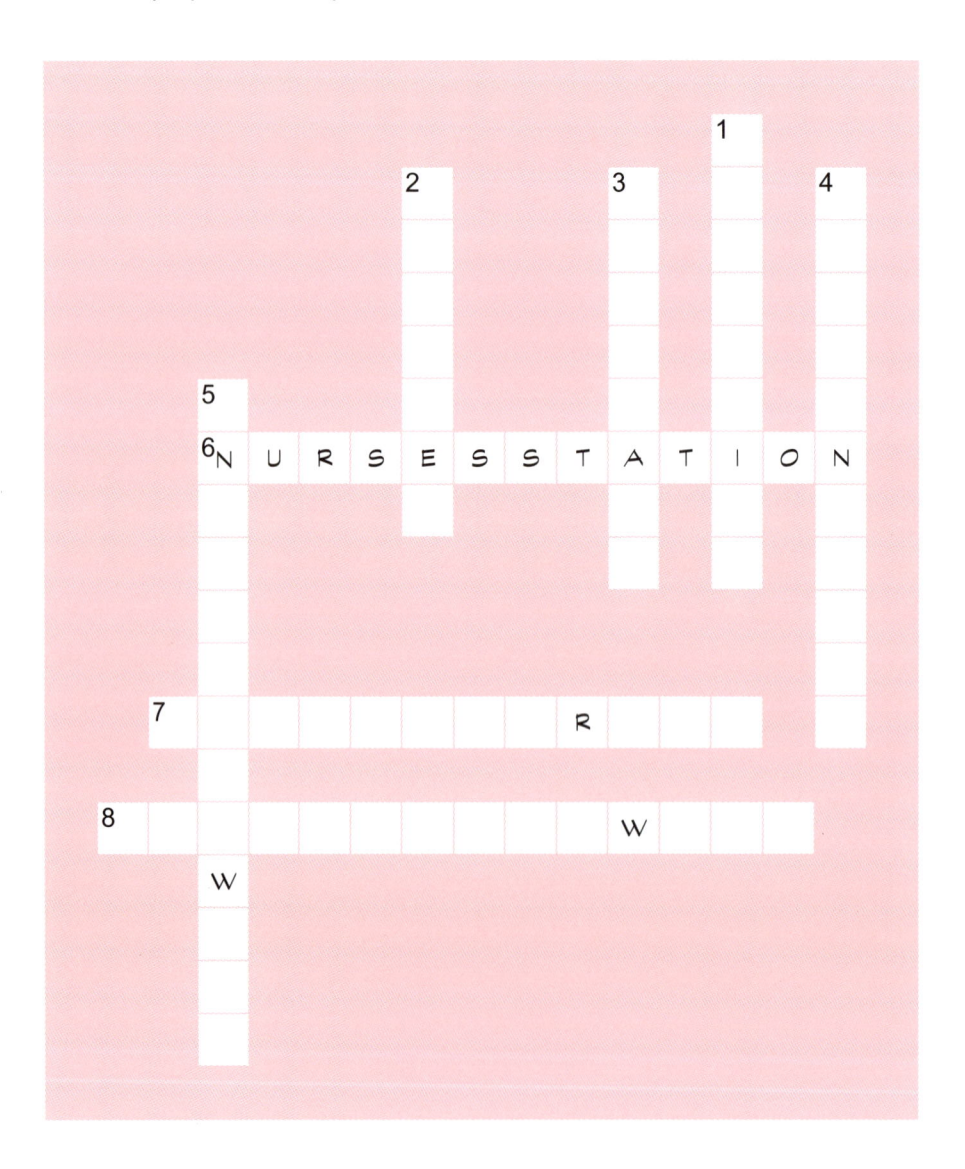

6. NURSESSTATION
7. _ _ _ _ _ _ _ R _ _ _
8. _ _ _ _ _ _ _ _ W _ _ _

パズルの鍵

ACROSS

6. An area in a hospital that serves as the center for patient nursing care.
7. A place where people first wake up after an operation.
8. An area of the hospital to treat sick people who are coming from outside and not staying overnight.

DOWN

1. A desk or area where visitors arriving at the hospital go first for registration.
2. A person or an area in the hospital where patients pay money for medical consultation, treatment, etc.
3. A store or a part of hospital where medicine is prepared and given out.
4. A place where people sit before seeing a doctor.
5. An area of the hospital which offers beds to sick people staying overnight for treatment.

［受付　待合室　薬局　会計　外来病棟　入院病棟　看護師詰め所　回復室］

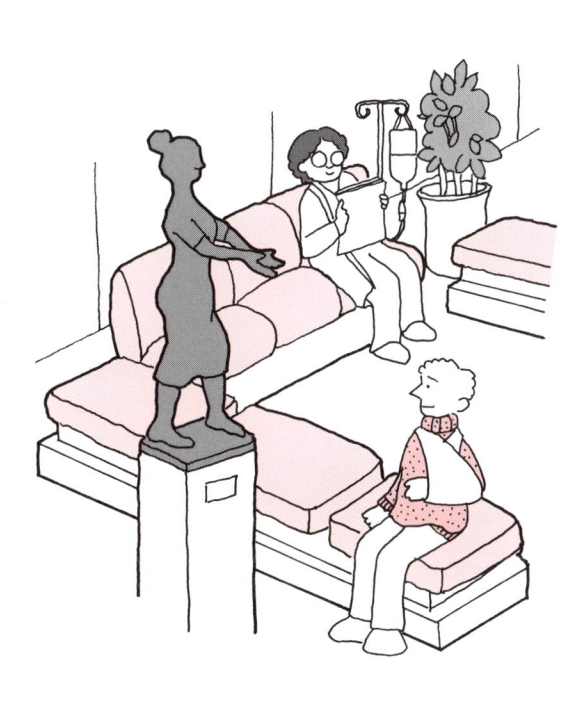

Chapter 6 The Elderly

Grandpa's Birthday

Story A

Hi Lotta,

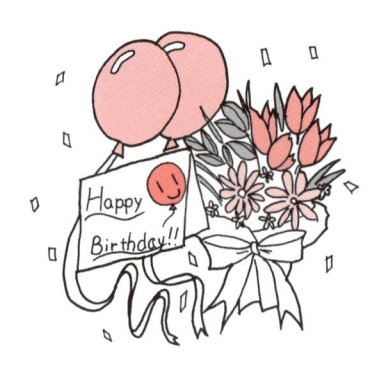

85歳のお誕生日おめでとう！

Yesterday was my grandfather's 85th birthday and all of our family visited Grandpa's senior facility to celebrate. Lotta, can you guess who joined us? It was Mats, who introduced you to me! When we met at the international festival, he told me that he was really interested in the Japanese way of life. That's why I invited him to our birthday visit.

Recently in Japan, the number of older parents living with children is decreasing, and many types of housing for the elderly are being developed. The place Grandpa lives in is an apartment offering various services to seniors. It is different from a normal apartment, and there is a large dining room, a common bath, a hobby room, a meeting room, etc.

Not only a manager but also nurses are on duty there. Each room has an emergency alarm for the residents to call staff members when they are not feeling well. Grandpa is a member of some clubs and enjoys light exercises or karaoke with other residents.

Grandpa regularly goes to a local senior day care center for rehabilitation. He sometimes visits the department of cardiology at a nearby hospital because of his heart problems. He is always smiling and telling jokes, so he is quite popular among the nurses and clinical staff there.

Word List

senior facility（2） 高齢者施設
Mats（3） ロッタの友人（Chapter 1 参照）
way of life（4） 暮らし方
birthday visit（5） 誕生日の訪問

housing for the elderly（7） 高齢者用住居
offering ～（8） ～を提供している
common bath（10） 共同浴場
hobby room（10） 娯楽室
meeting room（10） 集会室

on duty（11） 勤務している
when they are not feeling well（12） 具合が悪い時に
light exercise（13） 軽い体操
karaoke（14） カラオケ

senior day care center（15） 高齢者用デイケアセンター
department of cardiology（16） 循環器内科
clinical staff（18） 医療スタッフ

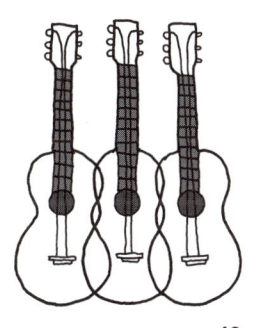

Chapter 6

Dialog 11 （診療科）

Nurse: Which department are you going to today?
Patient: I'm going to internal medicine.
Nurse: Please turn right at the first corner.
Patient: Thank you.

☆ 2人1組になってDialogを練習しましょう。交代して両方の役を行います。
☆ P.51のStep Up! Vocabularyを参考にして，下の会話を英語で行いましょう。
　そのほかの単語にも入れ替えて練習しましょう。

1. A：今日は何科に行かれますか？
   B：循環器内科に行きます。
   A：それではまっすぐ行って2つめの角を左に曲がってください。
   B：ありがとうございます。

2. A：今日は何科に行かれますか？
   B：整形外科に行きます。
   A：それでは2階に行ってください。
   B：ありがとうございます。

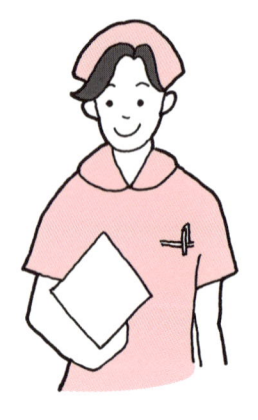

何科に行かれますか？

Step Up! Vocabulary

診療科　Department of...

- [ ] internal medicine
- [ ] cardiology
- [ ] respiratory medicine
- [ ] gastroenterology
- [ ] neurology
- [ ] surgery
- [ ] orthopedics
- [ ] plastic surgery
- [ ] urology
- [ ] radiology
- [ ] pediatrics
- [ ] obstetrics
- [ ] gynecology
- [ ] psychiatry
- [ ] dermatology
- [ ] ophthalmology
- [ ] oto (rhino) laryngology, ENT
- [ ] dentistry

- [ ] 内科
- [ ] 循環器内科
- [ ] 呼吸器内科
- [ ] 消化器内科
- [ ] 神経内科
- [ ] 外科
- [ ] 整形外科
- [ ] 形成外科
- [ ] 泌尿器科
- [ ] 放射線科
- [ ] 小児科
- [ ] 産科
- [ ] 婦人科
- [ ] 精神科
- [ ] 皮膚科
- [ ] 眼科
- [ ] 耳鼻（咽喉）科
- [ ] 歯科

院内の職業　Hospital Occupations

- [ ] nurse
- [ ] nurse's aide
- [ ] nursing student / student nurse
- [ ] midwife
- [ ] doctor
- [ ] resident
- [ ] clinical psychologist
- [ ] X-ray technician
- [ ] laboratory [lab] technician
- [ ] occupational therapist [OT]
- [ ] physical therapist [PT]
- [ ] speech therapist [ST]
- [ ] pharmacist
- [ ] dietitian
- [ ] (medical) social worker

- [ ] 看護師
- [ ] 看護助手
- [ ] 看護学生
- [ ] 助産師
- [ ] 医師
- [ ] レジデント，研修医
- [ ] 臨床心理士
- [ ] 放射線技師
- [ ] 検査技師
- [ ] 作業療法士
- [ ] 理学療法士
- [ ] 言語療法士
- [ ] 薬剤師
- [ ] 栄養士
- [ ] （医療）ソーシャルワーカー

Chapter 6
Story B

Grandpa really enjoyed our visit. We brought him his favorite Japanese traditional sweet called *yokan*. It is really sweet and Mats liked it very much. Lotta, I wonder if you would like it? Please give it a try if you come to Japan.

Grandpa is spending a peaceful life supported by family and the staff members of the senior facility. On the other hand, I hear that many elderly have problems because of physical or financial circumstances and a lack of facilities able to receive them. I hope in Japan more research and development will be done to support the elderly.

These days, Grandpa does not look in very good shape. When I was younger, he took me to many fun places, and I have a lot of good memories. I always hope he will stay healthy and live long.

The life span for Japanese men is 79 years and 86 for Japanese women, making average life expectancy for Japanese one of the highest in the world. Sweden is also one such country, isn't it? I hear that Sweden's welfare system is advanced and gives a comfortable life to the elderly and to people with disabilities. Lotta, do you also feel this way about Sweden's welfare system, and are you satisfied with it?

Hana

Word List

Japanese traditional sweet（1） 伝統的な和菓子
yokan（2） ようかん
give it a try（3） 試しに食べてみる

peaceful life（4） 穏やかな生活
on the other hand（5） 一方で
a lack of ～（6） ～の不足
able to receive ～（7） ～を受け入れる
research and development（7） 研究開発

in good shape（9） 体調がいい
fun place（10） 楽しい場所
stay healthy（11） 健康でいる

life span（12） 寿命
79 years and 86（12） （男性は）79歳で（女性は）86歳（2009年現在）
average life expectancy（13） 平均寿命

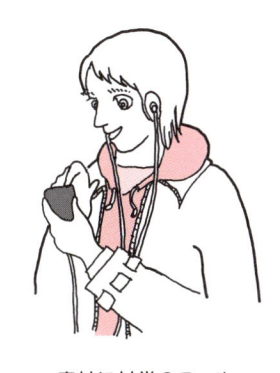

意外に甘党のマツツ

Chapter 6

Exercises

Ⅰ．本文の内容について正しい答えを選びましょう。

1. Who is working at Grandpa's senior facility?
   (a) a physical therapist and a nurse
   (b) an occupational therapist and a doctor
   (c) a manager and nurses
   (d) a manager and a doctor

2. What is in each room at Grandpa's senior facility?
   (a) an emergency alarm   (b) an emergency exit
   (c) emergency drugs   (d) emergency lights

3. Which department does Grandpa sometimes visit?
   (a) orthopedics   (b) pediatrics   (c) urology   (d) cardiology

Ⅱ．本文の内容に合うように（　）内の語順を入れ替えて英文を作りましょう。

1. 子どもと同居する高齢の親の数は減ってきている。

   The number (decreasing, living, of, older, children, parents, with, is).

2. 祖父は地域の高齢者デイケアセンターに定期的に通っている。

   (Grandpa, senior, a, day, care, goes, to, center, local) regularly.

Ⅲ．該当する診療科名を右から選びましょう。

1. dermatology   (　)   (a) 内科
2. radiology   (　)   (b) 歯科
3. plastic surgery (　)   (c) 皮膚科
4. dentistry   (　)   (d) 婦人科
5. internal medicine (　)   (e) 放射線科
6. gynecology   (　)   (f) 形成外科

Speaking Tips!

● 日本の食事を英語で説明するには？

もし外国人患者から病院食の内容を尋ねられたら，日本独特の食べ物はどう説明したらいいでしょうか。たとえば本文に出てくる「ようかん」は，"sweet bean jelly"と説明できそうです。では，次の食べ物は何でしょうか？　下の選択肢から選んでみましょう。

1. (　　) a bowl of cooked rice with beef
2. (　　) potatoes and meat stewed in soy sauce and sugar
3. (　　) boiled spinach with sesame dressing
4. (　　) steamed egg custard
5. (　　) grated Japanese radish
6. (　　) dried bonito flakes
7. (　　) devil's tongue〔a jelly-like food made from a kind of potato〕
8. (　　) steamed fish paste
9. (　　) rice cake
10. (　　) tofu〔soybean curd〕
11. (　　) miso〔soybean paste〕soup
12. (　　) fermented soybeans
13. (　　) pickled plums
14. (　　) green tea
15. (　　) barley tea

(A) 肉じゃが　(B) 牛丼　(C) 納豆　(D) 茶碗蒸し　(E) 麦茶　(F) みそ汁
(G) だいこんおろし　(H) こんにゃく　(I) かまぼこ　(J) 緑茶　(K) 餅
(L) 豆腐　(M) 梅干　(N) かつお節　(O) ほうれん草のごまあえ

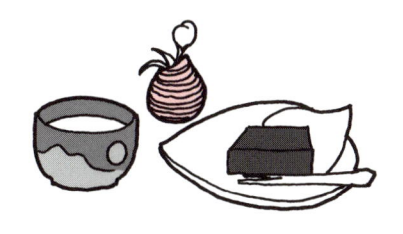

（解答は P.113）

Chapter 7 The Elderly

Grandma's House

おばあちゃんのお気に入り
森の中の小さな家

Story A

Hi Hana,

I'm glad that you and your family had a nice birthday with Mats. My grandmother is 87 years old, but still lives alone in her favorite small red house in the forest.

She uses elderly home care services, so visiting nurses or home care workers come daily to help her. The nurses help with medical care, and the home care workers assist with Grandma's cooking, cleaning, laundry, bathing, shopping, or sometimes just going for a walk. Thanks to such help, she can continue the lifestyle she has chosen for herself.

During the weekends, my parents or relatives visit her in turns to help out. My mother is in a "work sharing program" where she works three weeks and then gets one week off. During her break, she stays at Grandma's house to help her. In Sweden, the social welfare system may be advanced, but family support is also important. I love to visit her lovely old house—I always enjoy picking blueberries or mushrooms in the forest for her.

Of course some people prefer living in special senior apartments for self-supporting elderly. Others may want to live in "elderly homes" for people who need more daily assistance. We also have "nursing homes" with high-level medical care which treat elderly people with chronic illnesses. Another type of housing is "group homes" specializing in dementia care, shared by about five or six elderly people.

Word List

favorite small red house（2） お気に入りの小さな赤い家

elderly home care services（4） 高齢者の在宅ケアサービス
visiting nurse（4） 訪問看護師
home care worker（5） 訪問介護員，ホームヘルパー

work sharing program（10） ワークシェアリング*
one week off（11） 1週間の休み
pick blueberries or mushrooms（14） ブルーベリーやきのこを採る**

self-supporting elderly（16） 自立している高齢者
elderly home（16） 老人ホーム
nursing home（17） ナーシングホーム***
chronic illness（18） 慢性疾患
group home（19） グループホーム
dementia care（19） 認知症の介護

　＊ワークシェアリング…雇用確保・労働時間短縮などのために1つの仕事を2人以上で分け合う方式。
　＊＊スウェーデンには「自然享受権」という権利があり，個人で楽しむ限りは他人の所有する森や湖に入って果実を摘んだりできる。自然はみんなのものという考え。
＊＊＊ナーシングホーム…老人ホームより介護度が高く長期療養が必要な高齢者の住居。

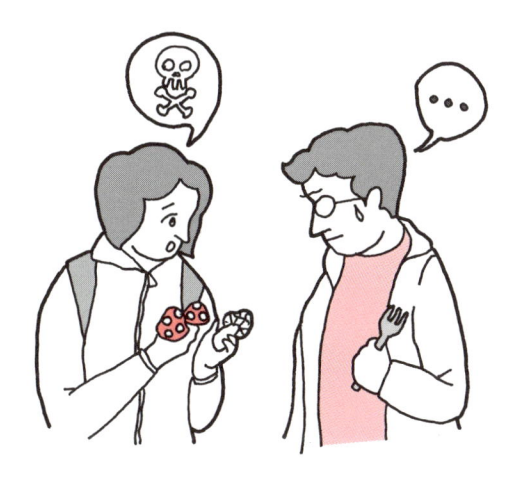

森できのこ狩り
毒きのこじゃないよね…？

Chapter 7

Dialog 12（日常の健康管理）

Visiting Nurse:　Do you have any health concerns?
Elderly Person:　I can't sleep well.
Visiting Nurse:　How many hours did you sleep last night?
Elderly Person:　Three hours.

☆　2人1組になってDialogを練習しましょう。交代して両方の役を行います。
☆　P. 59のStep Up! Vocabularyを参考にして，下の会話を英語で行いましょう。
　　そのほかの単語にも入れ替えて練習しましょう。

1. A：何か健康上のご心配がありますか？
   B：何度もトイレに行かないといけません。
   A：今日は何回おしっこに行きましたか？
   B：10回です。

2. A：何か健康上のご心配がありますか？
   B：食欲がありません。
   A：昨日は何回便通がありましたか？
   B：ありませんでした（none）。

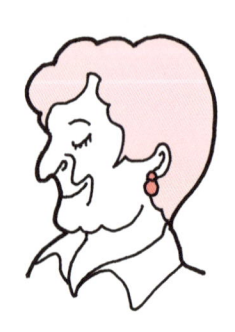

おばあちゃんは
いつだってステキ

Step Up! Vocabulary

日常の健康管理　Basic Daily Health Check

睡眠　Sleeping
- ☐ sleep
- ☐ sleeplessness, insomnia
- ☐ sleep disorder
- ☐ sleeping pill

- ☐ 睡眠，眠る
- ☐ 不眠
- ☐ 睡眠障害
- ☐ 睡眠薬

食事　Eating
- ☐ appetite
- ☐ appetite loss
- ☐ eating disorder
- ☐ swallowing disorder
- ☐ vomit, throw up
- ☐ burp

- ☐ 食欲
- ☐ 食欲不振
- ☐ 摂食障害
- ☐ 嚥下障害
- ☐ 嘔吐する
- ☐ ゲップ，ゲップをする

- ☐ food allergy
- ☐ vegetarian
- ☐ caloric restriction
- ☐ salt restriction
- ☐ protein restriction
- ☐ fluid restriction

- ☐ 食物アレルギー
- ☐ 菜食主義者，ベジタリアン
- ☐ カロリー制限
- ☐ 塩分制限
- ☐ タンパク制限
- ☐ 水分制限

排泄　Excretion
- ☐ urine
- ☐ urinate
- ☐ urination
- ☐ frequent urination
- ☐ bloody urine
- ☐ incontinence
- ☐ stool
- ☐ bowel movement
- ☐ have a bowel movement
- ☐ constipation
- ☐ diarrhea
- ☐ bloody stool

- ☐ 尿
- ☐ 排尿する
- ☐ 排尿
- ☐ 頻尿
- ☐ 血尿
- ☐ 失禁
- ☐ 便
- ☐ 排便，便通
- ☐ 排便する
- ☐ 便秘
- ☐ 下痢
- ☐ 血便

Chapter 7
Story B

Nowadays, we call various types of places for the elderly not "facilities" but "housing," aiming for a more homelike environment where each person's self-determination is respected.

The attached picture looks like a castle, but in reality it is a housing complex for the elderly. The rooms are often decorated with residents' favorite furniture and many photos full of nice memories. In some elderly housing, pets are welcomed to live with the elderly so that people can live a lifestyle they are used to. Other housing has restaurants open to the public to encourage exchanges between different generations.

In order to provide such varied care, taxes in Sweden are very high. Sales tax is 25% and it is not unusual to pay half of one's income in taxes. However, it is said that 75% of taxes we pay come back to us in welfare services like medical care, assistance in raising children and support for the elderly.

I think that this system shows our country's fundamental attitude to people's welfare—any risks that occur in one's life must be shared by society as a whole, so as not to leave the responsibility to the individual or family alone. Hana, you asked me if I am satisfied with the social welfare system of this country. Well, I believe that this welfare system is one which we can be proud of, although we are still continuing to improve it.

Lotta

Word List

various types of places for the elderly（1） さまざまな高齢者住居（Story A 第4段落参照）
not "facilities" but "housing"（1） 「施設」でなく「住居」
aiming for ～（2） ～を目標に
self-determination（3） 自己決定

housing complex（4） 複合住宅
live a lifestyle they are used to（7） 以前の生活と同じような暮らし方をする
exchanges between different generations（9） 異世代間の交流

sales tax（10） 消費税
in taxes（11） 税金に
assistance in raising children（13） 子育て支援

fundamental attitude（14） 基本的な姿勢
occur in one's life（15） 人生に起こる
by society as a whole（15） 社会全体で
so as not to leave the responsibility to the individual or family alone（16）
　　個人や家族だけに責任を負わせないように
one which we can be proud of（18） 私たちが自慢できるものの1つ

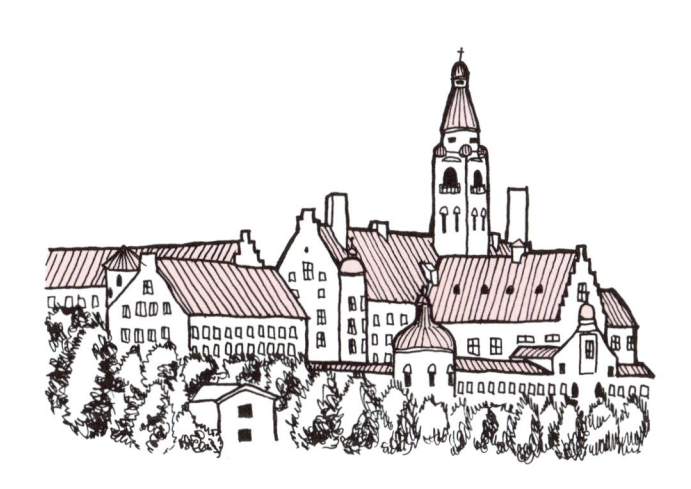

どう見てもお城だけど…

Chapter 7

Exercises

Ⅰ. 本文の内容について正しい答えを選びましょう。

1. How often does Lotta's mother go to help Grandma?
   (a) every day　　(b) every week
   (c) every month　(d) every other month

2. How much is the sales tax in Sweden according to Lotta's explanation?
   (a) 10%　(b) 15%　(c) 25%　(d) 50%

3. What is Lotta's feeling about the Swedish social welfare system?
   (a) It is not very good and needs much more improvement.
   (b) It is good but needs more improvement.
   (c) It is very good and does not need more improvement.

Ⅱ. 本文中で次の高齢者用住居はどのように説明されていますか。ふさわしいものを選択肢から選びましょう。

1. group home (　　)　2. nursing home (　　)　3. elderly home (　　)

   (a) housing for elderly people who need more daily assistance than self-supporting people
   (b) housing for elderly people who need special dementia care in a shared house
   (c) housing for elderly people with chronic illnesses who need high-level medical care

Ⅲ. 該当する日本語を右から選びましょう。

1. sleeping pill　　　(　　)　(a) 睡眠障害
2. fluid restriction　(　　)　(b) 摂食障害
3. constipation　　　(　　)　(c) 食欲不振
4. eating disorder　 (　　)　(d) 睡眠薬
5. sleep disorder　　(　　)　(e) 便秘
6. appetite loss　　　(　　)　(f) 水分制限

Reading Tips!

● **ロイヤル・ファミリーと社会福祉**

スウェーデン国王一家の居城の近くに,「シルビアホーム」という認知症高齢者専門センターがあります。シルビア王妃の母親がアルツハイマー病を患った経験から,王妃自身が提唱し,1995年に設立されました。緑豊かな場所にあるとても家族的な雰囲気のところで,「シルビアシスター」(男性でも)という専門資格をもった介護スタッフがケアを行っています。広々としたサンルームで木々の揺らぎを眺めながらのティータイムや音楽など,ゆったりとした時間が流れています。

また,次の国王になる長女のビクトリアは,「ビクトリア・ローズ」という名前のバラの花を売った収益を障がいや病気をもつ子どもたちに寄付するなど,福祉を充実させるためのさまざまな活動を積極的に行っています。

● **夏休みは5週間**

北国スウェーデンの人々が1年で一番楽しみにしているのは,6月から始まる夏の休暇かもしれません。たっぷり5週間取れるので,家族で森や湖や小さな島などにある簡素なサマーハウスに行き,自然の中でのんびり日光浴をしたり,本を読んだりして暮らします。

日頃はバリバリのビジネスマンでEメールの返事をこまめに返してくれる人も,この期間はぷっつり音信不通になったりします。「サマーハウスにはインターネットの設備がないから」と,メールの返事が1か月以上経ってから返って来ることも。なお,郵便物はこの期間,サマーハウスに転送してもらうこともできるそうです。国をあげて夏休みを大切にしているのは,ちょっぴりうらやましい気がします。

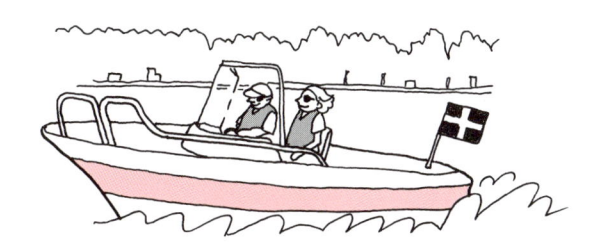

Word Search 2　院内の職業

```
E K Q Y U B Z A C X B R K N V
V M C E N A I T I T E I D U K
O X I M Y L O V E K X O K R A
I O F D K P H A R M A C I S T
R U G R W J E O C E V R C E I
J Y A J Z I W Z A I W H E D Z
W E O H K L F O F K E C O X F
H Q B J A R U E Q G Z C G K Q
U N A I C I N H C E T B A L E
F T C H O W O A V O A R U G Y
Y O I X A I Y K R E W V Q O A
S P E E C H T H E R A P I S T
A F G O O D L U C K H I G J C
K E Z T R F C E Q Y W H U A V
I Q J A B W T H G K E B T R F
```

☆　上の表の中に病院内のさまざまな職業の名前がタテ・ヨコ・ナナメに隠れています。探して丸で囲みましょう。また，各語を日本語で書きましょう。

1. nurse　　　　　(　　　　　)　　5. dietitian　　　　(　　　　　)
2. midwife　　　　(　　　　　)　　6. pharmacist　　　(　　　　　)
3. doctor　　　　(　　　　　)　　7. speech therapist (　　　　　)
4. lab technician (　　　　　)　　8. social worker　　(　　　　　)

Game 2　道案内ゲーム　"Can you tell me the way?"

☆ 教室のどこか好きな場所に，カバンやペンケースなど「ターゲット」になるものを1つ置きます。先生か学生が1人，教室の入口に立って患者役になります。ほかの学生たちは順番に（座席順など）英語で指示をして，ターゲットを手に入れられるように道案内をしましょう。

（下図の例）　① Go straight.　② Stop.　　　③ Turn left.　　④ Go forward.
　　　　　　　⑤ Stop.　　　　⑥ Turn right.　⑦ Go straight.

時には，わざと違う指示をしてもかまいません。

（例）　Turn around. / Go back. / Don't turn left.

慣れてきたら目標物を2個以上にして，それぞれ離れた場所に置き，全部回収できるまで英語で道案内をしましょう。

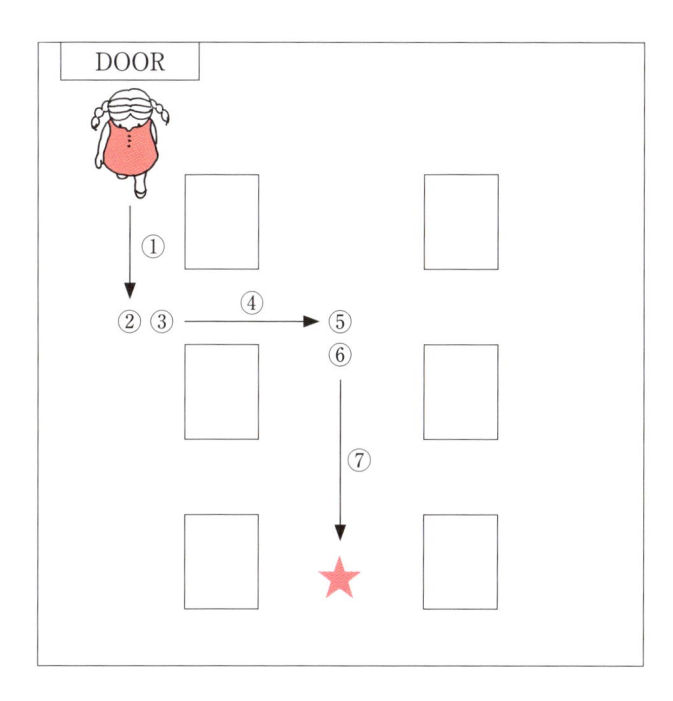

Chapter 8 People with Disabilities

Living Independently

Story A

Hi Lotta,

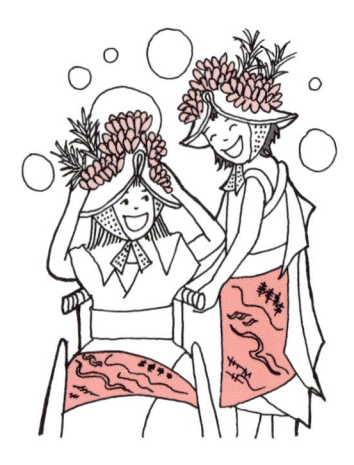

ハナちゃん、一緒に踊ろう！

Today, I'd like to tell you about my best friend Yuki. Ever since she was in a traffic accident, she has been in a wheelchair but always keeps a positive attitude. Yuki and I often enjoy talking about many things, including secret loves!

Yuki's morning begins at 7:30 a.m. with a visit from a home care worker who helps her to get dressed and prepare breakfast. Home care workers also come at dinner and before bedtime. The types of care she needs are physical care, housework and help when going out.

She has contracts with three home care providers and employs a total of eight people to assist her. In the past, she did not have the freedom to choose her own home care workers. They were sent by the authorities and so people with disabilities felt in a weak position always asking for help. However, under the new system, she is able to freely choose home care workers, and hire them according to what the system allows her.

The Japanese system classifies people who have disabilities from levels 1 to 6 according to their conditions. The amount of benefits a person can receive depends on the disability level. Payments for care vary according to the individual income level. For example, Yuki pays 10% of the total care costs.

Word List

ever since ~（1） ～以来ずっと
(be) in a traffic accident（1） 交通事故に遭う
(be) in a wheelchair（2） 車いすで生活している
keep a positive attitude（2） 前向きな姿勢でいる
secret love（3） 内緒の恋（人）

physical care（7） 身体介護
help when going out（8） 外出支援

home care provider（9） 在宅介護事業者
the authorities（11） 行政当局
weak position（12） 弱い立場
always asking for help（12） いつも助けを求めるばかりの
according to what the system allows her（14） 制度で認められた範囲内で

benefit（16） 支援・特典
individual income level（18） それぞれの収入の度合い

Chapter 8

Dialog 13（日常生活動作）

Nurse: Can you eat by yourself?
Patient: Yes, I can.
Nurse: Can you walk by yourself?
Patient: Yes, but I need a cane.

☆ 2人1組になってDialogを練習しましょう。交代して両方の役を行います。
☆ P. 69のStep Up! Vocabularyを参考にして，下の会話を英語で行いましょう。
そのほかの単語にも入れ替えて練習しましょう。

1. A：自分で洋服を着られますか？
   B：はい，できます。
   A：自分で階段を上れますか？
   B：はい。でも手すりが必要です。

2. A：自分で歩けますか？
   B：いいえ。車いすが必要です。
   A：自分で入浴できますか？
   B：いいえ。介助（help）が必要です。

Step Up! Vocabulary

日常生活動作　Activities of Daily Living [ADL]

- ☐ walk
- ☐ stand up
- ☐ sit down
- ☐ go up [down] stairs
- ☐ transfer to [from] a wheelchair [a bed]
- ☐ sit up
- ☐ roll over
- ☐ eat
- ☐ drink water
- ☐ take medicine
- ☐ urinate*
- ☐ have a bowel movement*
- ☐ dress / undress
- ☐ brush one's teeth
- ☐ wash one's face [body] [hair]
- ☐ comb one's hair

- ☐ 歩く
- ☐ 立ち上がる
- ☐ 座る
- ☐ 階段を上る〔下りる〕
- ☐ 車いす〔ベッド〕に〔から〕移る
- ☐ 起き上がる（寝ている状態から）
- ☐ 寝返りを打つ
- ☐ 食べる
- ☐ 水を飲む
- ☐ 薬を飲む
- ☐ 排尿する
- ☐ 排便する
- ☐ 服を着る / 脱ぐ
- ☐ 歯を磨く
- ☐ 顔〔体〕〔髪〕を洗う
- ☐ 整髪する

生活補助手段　Assisted Living Equipment and Methods

- ☐ hearing aid
- ☐ magnifying glass
- ☐ reading machine
- ☐ (white) cane
- ☐ quad cane
- ☐ crutch(es)
- ☐ walker
- ☐ wheelchair
- ☐ handrail
- ☐ wheelchair ramp
- ☐ stair lift
- ☐ Braille**
- ☐ textured paving block(s)
- ☐ service [assistance] dog
- ☐ sign language

- ☐ 補聴器
- ☐ 拡大鏡
- ☐ 読書機
- ☐ （白）杖
- ☐ 4点ステッキ
- ☐ 松葉杖
- ☐ 歩行器
- ☐ 車いす
- ☐ 手すり
- ☐ 車いす用スロープ
- ☐ 階段用リフト，昇降機
- ☐ 点字
- ☐ 点字ブロック
- ☐ 介助犬
- ☐ 手話

＊Chapter 7 既出　＊＊発案者の人名（ルイ・ブライユ）に由来

Chapter 8

Story B

Awareness about a "barrier-free society" and "universal design" is gradually increasing in Japan. We now see various devices to help people with disabilities, such as textured paving blocks or wheelchair ramps. New buildings are often designed to be easily accessible for everybody.

These days, the number of buses that can take wheelchairs is increasing, but in reality it's difficult for wheelchairs to enter buses that are always crowded. In Japan, it is still challenging for people with disabilities to get around town.

In spite of this, my friend Yuki doesn't stay quietly at home. She works at the reception desk of a hospital. I like to see her moving freely around the hospital in her wheelchair and enjoying her work. However, Yuki says it is still really difficult for people with disabilities to find work.

Yuki also does other activities with a positive attitude as much as she can. When she attended a Japanese festival supported by volunteers, she enjoyed dancing with me wearing a traditional costume! Please look at the picture. It's beautiful, isn't it?

Previously in Japan, usually only protective care was provided to people with disabilities. However, nowadays, there are many additional programs to encourage them to live more independently. Since there are many disabled people with various talents, I think that we must continue to develop a society where these people can contribute.

Hana

Living Independently

Word List

awareness（1） 意識，自覚
barrier-free（1） バリアフリー
universal design（1） ユニバーサルデザイン
textured paving block（3） 点字ブロック
wheelchair ramp（3） 車いす用スロープ
easily accessible for everybody（4） 誰でも利用しやすい

buses that can take wheelchairs（5） 車いすで乗れるバス
it is still challenging（7） まだ簡単ではない
get around town（7） 街に出かける

stay quietly at home（8） ひっそり家に閉じこもる
move freely around the hospital（9） 院内を自由に動き回る

traditional costume（14） 伝統的な（民族）衣装

protective care（16） 保護的なケア
many additional（17） さらに多くの
society where these people can contribute（19） このような人々が貢献できる社会

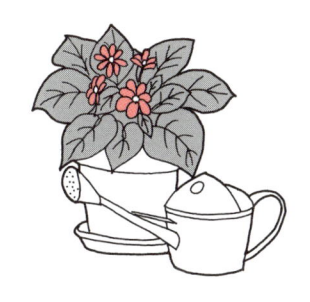

ユキちゃんは
花を育てるのが好き

Chapter 8

Exercises

Ⅰ．本文の内容と一致するものには○，そうでないものには×をつけましょう。

1. （　　）Yuki has contracts with three home care providers but does not have the freedom to choose her own home care workers.
2. （　　）The types of care Yuki needs are physical care, housework and help when going out.
3. （　　）In Japan, it is still challenging for people with disabilities to get around town because there are not enough buses that can take wheelchairs.
4. （　　）Hana thinks that the Japanese social welfare system is gradually developing.
5. （　　）In the Japanese system, people with disabilities are divided into five levels according to their conditions.

Ⅱ．本文の内容に合うように（　　　　）内の語順を入れ替えて英文を作りましょう。

1. 日本ではバリアフリー社会についての意識が高まってきている。

  （about, increasing, a barrier-free society, awareness, is）in Japan.

2. 彼女はボランティアに支えられて日本の祭に参加した。

  （by, Japanese, a, festival, she, volunteers, attended, supported）.

Ⅲ．該当する日本語を右から選びましょう。

1. crutch(es)　　　（　　）　(a) 補聴器
2. hearing aid　　　（　　）　(b) 白杖
3. sign language　　（　　）　(c) 松葉杖
4. walker　　　　　（　　）　(d) 拡大鏡
5. magnifying glass （　　）　(e) 手話
6. white cane　　　（　　）　(f) 歩行器

Reading Tips!

● 「障がい者」を英語で何と言う？

障がいをもつ人のことを英語でどう言えばいいのでしょうか？ 以前は"handicapped"という語が使われることが多かったのですが，今ではこれはあまり適切でないと考えられています。その理由には諸説ありますが，語源に否定的な意味があるとも言われています。

本書では，英字新聞等によく用いられる"people with disabilities"という言い方を主に使っています。

さらに，"person(s) with disabilities"のほうが，より好ましいと言う人もいます。1人ひとり個別の人格なのに障がいをもつという点だけで全員を"people"とひとまとめにするよりも，"person"という個人を対象にするほうがよい，という考えです。

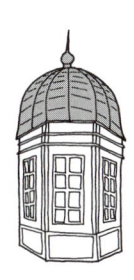

最近では"challenged,""differently-abled,""less able-bodied"という言い方が使われることもありますが，賛否両論です。英語の表現も常に移り変わっていきます。

Chapter 9 People with Disabilities

Everyone is Different

Story A

Hi Hana,

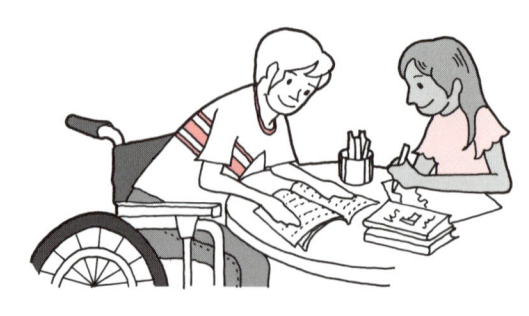

ねえ，これおもしろいよ！

Today, I will write about the school where I work. The school is located in the northern part of the city surrounded by beautiful nature. We often go to a nearby forest and lake for classes.

The school has 300 students ranging from 6 to 14 years of age. Among these students, 50 children have minor to more serious disabilities. Our aim is to have an inclusive school where students with and without disabilities study together.

Yesterday we had our annual sports day. We planned the events carefully so that all the students could take part. Adam won the gold medal in a walking race. He is twelve years old and has hearing problems because he had meningitis when he was young. Adam looked very happy and proud of his achievement.

Our role in the school is to encourage the students to increase their self-confidence and independence. In order to achieve this, we give them as many chances as possible during their school days. We always help them reach their potential and try not to help them too much. Our goal is that people, with and without disabilities, can live "normal" and happy lives, making the most of their own abilities.

Word List

for classes（3） 授業のために

minor to more serious disabilities（5） 軽度からより重度の障がい
inclusive（6） 包括的な*

take part（9） 参加する
has hearing problems（10） 聴力に問題がある
meningitis（11） 髄膜炎
when he was young（11） 幼い時に
achievement（12） （努力して）達成したこと

increase self-confidence and independence（13） 自信と自立心を育てる
reach potential（16） 潜在能力を発揮する
"normal" life（17） 「普通の」生活**
make the most of their own abilities（18） 自分自身の能力を最大限に生かす

＊インクルージョン（包括教育）…障がいのある子に限らず子どもは最初から1人ずつ違う特性をもつ存在と考え，それぞれのニーズに応じた教育支援を行うこと。
＊＊ノーマライゼーション…障がいをもっていても区別されることなく，ほかの人と同じようにごく普通の生活を送ることを当然とする考え。1960年代に北欧から始まった。

Reading Tips!

● 学校はカラフル

日本の教室の内装は一般的に落ち着いた色調が使われていますが，スウェーデンの学校では鮮やかな色合いのインテリアをよく見かけます。生徒用の机が緑色でいすは赤だったり，大胆な花柄のカーテンがかけてあったりしますが，あちこちに飾られた花や絵や織物が調和して，全体がとても素敵に見えます。さすがインテリアの伝統ある国だからでしょうか。Chapter 2でご紹介した"Art in Hospital"もそうですが，家庭や学校，職場を問わず，人々が毎日を過ごすための環境をとても大事にする国だと思います。

Chapter 9

Dialog 14（病歴）

Nurse: Have you ever had a serious disease?
Patient: I had meningitis when I was four years old.
Nurse: Do you have any problems now?
Patient: No, I'm fine now.

☆ 2人1組になってDialogを練習しましょう。交代して両方の役を行います。
☆ P. 80のStep Up! Vocabularyを参考に下の会話を英語で行いましょう。
そのほかの単語にも入れ替えて練習しましょう。

1. A：これまでに何か大きな病気をしたことがありますか？
   B：2年前に肺炎にかかりました。
   A：今は何か問題がありますか？
   B：いいえ，もう大丈夫です。

2. A：これまでに何か大きな病気をしたことがありますか？
   B：47歳の時に白血病にかかりました。
   A：今は何か問題がありますか？
   B：はい，今も治療中（receiving treatment）です。

Story B

I think that many kinds of disabilities only become apparent because of the environment, not because of the individual's physical condition. For example, wheelchair users can get around town by themselves, but cannot enter a building that has only stairs. If the environment can be made more accessible using various devices, inconveniences for people with disabilities will be minimized.

My country has various systems to provide services for individuals with different needs. For example, children with allergies are given specially cooked lunches at school. If there is a student from Japan, the school will look for a Japanese-speaking teacher and include a weekly class to maintain the student's native language ability.

People are different in some ways—physical appearance, health condition, ethnicity, etc. I think that disabilities can be one of those differences. Regardless of disabilities, I believe that everyone has the right to enjoy life and receive appropriate services for their condition.

I really love my job because I can help people overcome barriers and I am able to see the smiling faces of children everyday. Hana, please come to see our school someday and meet my lovely students.

Lotta

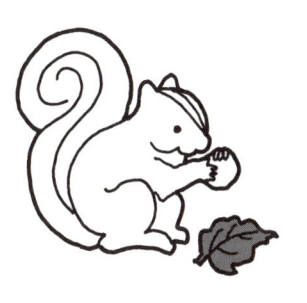

学校の庭には
リスもあそびに来ます

Chapter 9

Word List

only become apparent because of the environment（1）
　環境が原因となってはじめて表れる
individual's physical condition（2）　個人の身体状況
building that has only stairs（4）　階段しかない建物
if the environment can be made more accessible（4）
　もし環境（自体）を誰もがもっと利用しやすいように変えられれば
using various devices（5）　さまざまな工夫で
inconvenience（5）　不自由，困難
（be）minimized（5）　最小限になる，限りなく小さくなる

individuals with different needs（7）　さまざまなニーズをもつ1人ひとり
include a weekly class（10）　毎週の授業を組み込む

in some ways（12）　いろいろな意味で，いろいろな点で
physical appearance（12）　外見
ethnicity（13）　民族性
can be one of those differences（13）　そんな違いの1つと言える
regardless of disabilities（14）　障がい（の有無）にかかわらず
appropriate services for their condition（15）　それぞれの状態に応じた適切なサービス

overcome barriers（16）　障壁（となるもの）を乗り越える

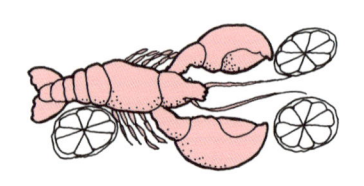

北欧の夏の風物詩
ザリガニパーティー

Exercises

Ⅰ. 本文の内容と一致するものには○，そうでないものには×をつけましょう。

1. (　　) The school where Lotta works has a total of 350 students with and without disabilities.
2. (　　) The school encourages the students to increase their self-confidence and independence.
3. (　　) Lotta thinks that people are different in some ways.
4. (　　) Lotta's country does not have various systems to provide services for individuals with different needs.
5. (　　) Japanese students can have special classes to maintain their native language ability at school.

Ⅱ. 本文の内容に合うように（　　）内の語順を入れ替えて文章を作りましょう。

1. 50人の子どもたちが軽度からより重度の障害をもっている。

    (children, more, disabilities, have, fifty, minor, to, serious).

2. アレルギーのある子どもたちは特別に調理した昼食が与えられる。

    (allergies, lunches, cooked, are, with, given, specially, children).

Ⅲ. 該当する日本語を右から選びましょう。

1.	hypertension	(　　)	(a) 気管支炎
2.	chickenpox	(　　)	(b) 肺炎
3.	mumps	(　　)	(c) 高血圧
4.	tetanus	(　　)	(d) 水ぼうそう
5.	measles	(　　)	(e) おたふく風邪
6.	fracture	(　　)	(f) 破傷風
7.	rubella	(　　)	(g) 麻疹
8.	sprain	(　　)	(h) 風疹
9.	bronchitis	(　　)	(i) 骨折
10.	pneumonia	(　　)	(j) ねんざ

Chapter 9

Step Up! Vocabulary

病名　Diseases

脳神経系

- ☐ stroke
    - ☐ cerebral infarction
    - ☐ cerebral hemorrhage
- ☐ Parkinson's disease
- ☐ Alzheimer's disease
- ☐ dementia
- ☐ epilepsy

- ☐ （脳）卒中
    - ☐ 脳梗塞
    - ☐ 脳出血
- ☐ パーキンソン病
- ☐ アルツハイマー病
- ☐ 認知症
- ☐ てんかん

循環器系

- ☐ heart attack
    - ☐ angina
    - ☐ myocardial infarction
- ☐ hypertension

- ☐ 心臓発作
    - ☐ 狭心症
    - ☐ 心筋梗塞
- ☐ 高血圧

呼吸器系

- ☐ bronchitis
- ☐ （bronchial）asthma
- ☐ pneumonia

- ☐ 気管支炎
- ☐ （気管支）喘息
- ☐ 肺炎

消化器系

- ☐ gastroenteritis
- ☐ gastric〔stomach〕ulcer
- ☐ duodenal ulcer
- ☐ appendicitis
- ☐ hepatitis A〔B〕〔C〕
- ☐ cirrhosis
- ☐ gallstone(s)
- ☐ pancreatitis

- ☐ 胃腸炎
- ☐ 胃潰瘍
- ☐ 十二指腸潰瘍
- ☐ 虫垂炎
- ☐ A〔B〕〔C〕型肝炎
- ☐ 肝硬変
- ☐ 胆石
- ☐ 膵炎

腎泌尿器系

- ☐ kidney stone(s)
- ☐ kidney failure

- ☐ 腎結石
- ☐ 腎不全

Everyone is Different

病名

代謝・内分泌系
- ☐ diabetes (mellitus) ☐ 糖尿病
- ☐ gout ☐ 痛風

感染症系
- ☐ common cold ☐ 風邪, 感冒
- ☐ influenza [flu] ☐ インフルエンザ
- ☐ tuberculosis ☐ 結核
- ☐ whooping cough, pertussis ☐ 百日咳
- ☐ diphtheria ☐ ジフテリア
- ☐ tetanus ☐ 破傷風
- ☐ measles ☐ 麻疹, はしか
- ☐ rubella ☐ 風疹
- ☐ chickenpox ☐ 水ぼうそう
- ☐ mumps ☐ おたふく風邪
- ☐ polio ☐ ポリオ, 小児まひ
- ☐ AIDS ☐ エイズ

その他
- ☐ cancer ☐ 悪性腫瘍, がん
- ☐ leukemia ☐ 白血病
- ☐ hives ☐ じんましん
- ☐ cataract ☐ 白内障
- ☐ tonsillitis ☐ 扁桃炎
- ☐ sinusitis ☐ 副鼻腔炎
- ☐ depression ☐ うつ病
- ☐ fracture ☐ 骨折
- ☐ sprain ☐ ねんざ

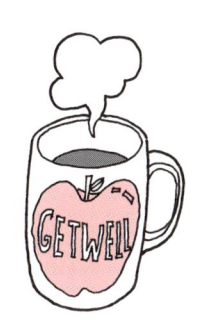

お大事に…

Crossword Puzzle 2　診療科

☆ 下の空欄には病院のいろいろな診療科名が入ります。ヒントの英文と［　　］内の選択肢を参考にして，空欄を英語で埋めましょう。難しい場合は Chapter 6 (P. 51) の Step Up! Vocabulary を参考にしましょう。

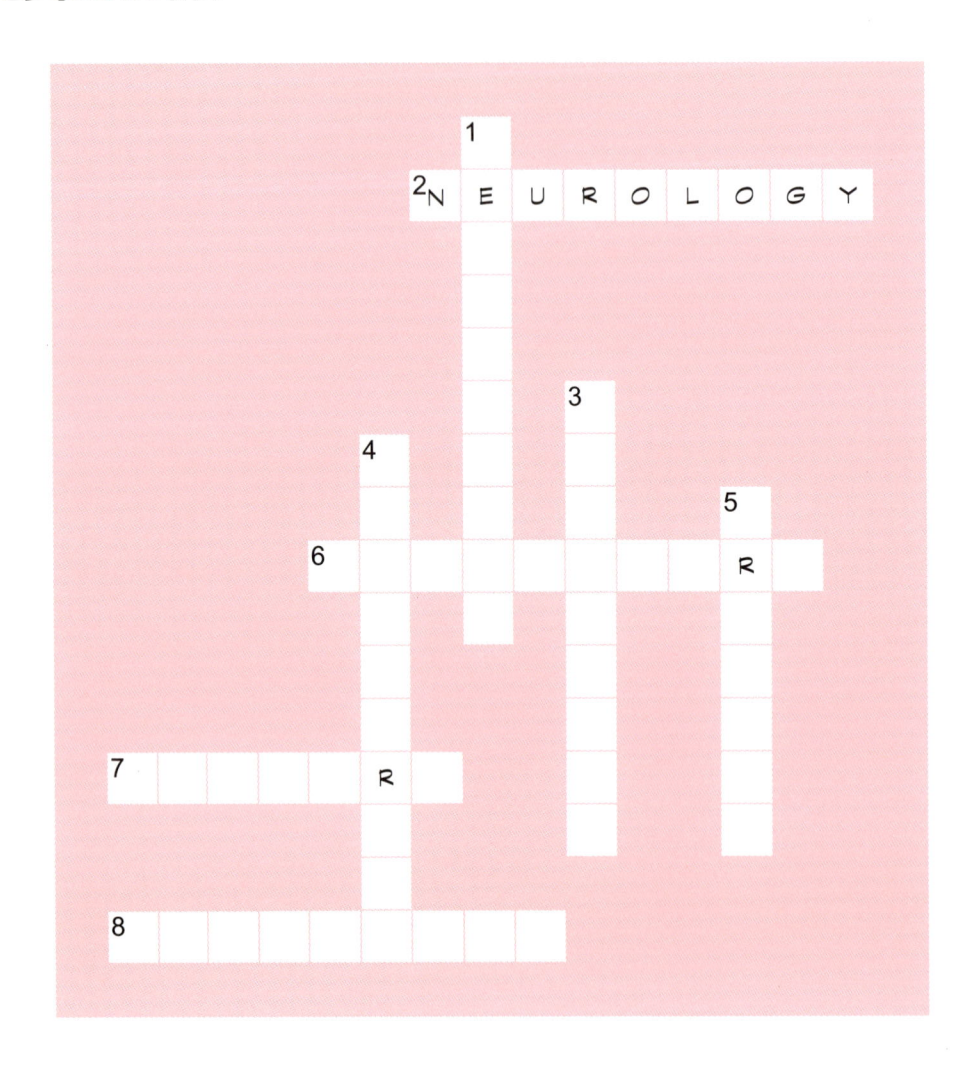

パズルの鍵

The area of medicine that deals with …

ACROSS
2. … the nervous system and its diseases.
6. … mental illnesses.
7. … treatment by cutting open the body.
8. … the teeth and the mouth.

DOWN
1. … children and their illnesses.
3. … medical use of radiation.
4. … the birth of children.
5. … the urinary system and male sexual organs.

［小児科　外科　産科　神経内科　泌尿器科　放射線科　精神科　歯科］

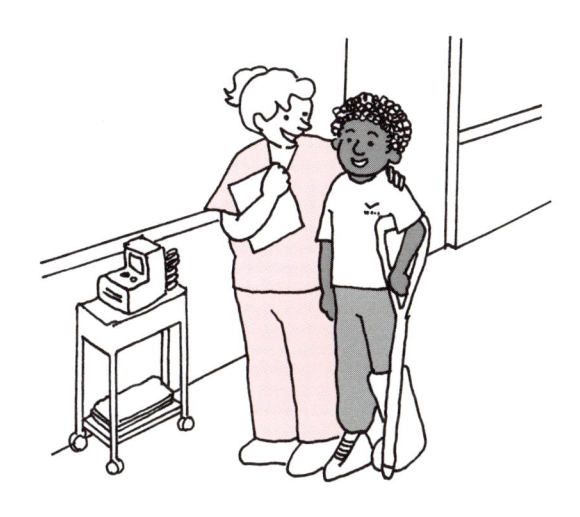

Chapter 10 A Nurse's Job

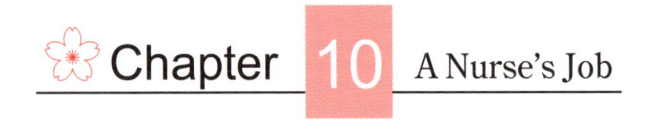

Hospital Training Begins

Story A

Hi Lotta,

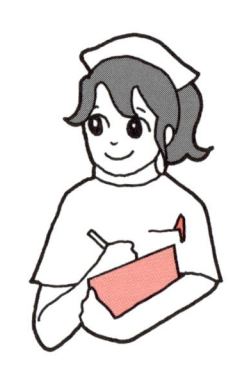

いよいよ看護実習！

Finally we have started nursing training at the hospital. The patient I'm caring for is a 29-year-old male who had a traffic accident. I'm wearing a white uniform and carrying a stethoscope which makes me feel like Nightingale! But honestly, taking care of a young man is a little embarrassing.

First, I distribute meals and help my patient to eat. Next, I check his temperature, pulse and blood pressure. Since I practiced this many times at school, everything is going smoothly.

Then I give him a bed bath. This is unexpectedly difficult as just touching the patient makes me feel nervous. I worry if the patient is uncomfortable or has pain because of my care. It takes a long time and I always end up in a nervous sweat.

Furthermore, I feel pressure from the senior nurses. When they are helping doctors to treat wounds by disinfecting and changing dressings, I don't know what to do and feel completely useless. Even though I was mentally prepared beforehand, the actual workplace is always stressful. The usual happy-go-lucky me is now feeling down....

Word List

hospital training　病院実習
nursing training（1）　看護実習
care for ～（2）　～のケアをする，世話をする
white uniform（3）　白衣
stethoscope（3）　聴診器
Nightingale（4）　ナイチンゲール＊

distribute meals（5）　食事の配膳をする
everything is going smoothly（7）　どれもうまくいっている

give a bed bath（8）　清拭(せいしき)する
feel nervous（9）　緊張する
worry if ～（9）　～ではないかと心配する
end up ～（10）　結局～になる
nervous sweat（10）　冷や汗

senior nurse（12）　先輩看護師
change dressings（13）　包帯交換をする
mentally prepared（14）　心の準備をしている
happy-go-lucky（16）　のんきな，楽天的な
feel down（16）　（気分が）落ち込む，しょんぼりする

＊フローレンス・ナイチンゲール（1820-1910）…英国の看護師。クリミア戦争で傷病兵の看護を献身的に行い，教育者としても近代看護の確立に貢献した。

Chapter 10

Dialog 15（治療・処置）

Nurse: I'll give you an injection.
Please make a fist.
Please open your hand.
Now it's over.

☆ 2人1組で看護師のセリフを練習しましょう。相手（患者役）に実際に話しかけるつもりで言いましょう。

☆ P. 87 の Step Up! Vocabulary を参考に下の看護師の会話を英語で言ってみましょう。そのほかの単語にも入れ替えて練習しましょう。

1. 点滴をします。
   動かないでください。

2. 浣腸をします。
   できるだけ（as ~ as possible）長くがまんして（hold it in）ください。

3. 傷を消毒します。
   少ししみる（sting）かもしれません。

4. 医師が鼻から（through your nose）挿管します。
   リラックスしてください。

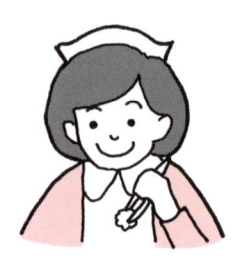

ちょっぴりしみますけど

Hospital Training Begins

Step Up! Vocabulary

治療・処置　Treatments

- ☐ injection, shot   ☐ 注射
- ☐ intravenous drip [IV]   ☐ 点滴
- ☐ blood transfusion   ☐ 輸血
- ☐ blood sampling   ☐ 採血
- ☐ disinfection   ☐ 消毒
- ☐ incision   ☐ 切開
- ☐ stitch, suture   ☐ 縫合
- ☐ stitch removal   ☐ 抜糸
- ☐ dressing change   ☐ 包帯交換
- ☐ anesthesia   ☐ 麻酔
- ☐ suction   ☐ 吸引
- ☐ intubation   ☐ 挿管
- ☐ urethral catheterization   ☐ 導尿
- ☐ enema   ☐ 浣腸
- ☐ bed bath   ☐ 清拭
- ☐ first aid   ☐ 応急処置

- ◇ give an injection [a shot]   ◇ 注射する
- ◇ give an IV   ◇ 点滴する
- ◇ give a blood transfusion   ◇ 輸血する
- ◇ take a blood sample   ◇ 採血する
- ◇ disinfect   ◇ 消毒する
- ◇ make an incision   ◇ 切開する
- ◇ stitch a wound   ◇ 縫合する
- ◇ remove stitches   ◇ 抜糸する
- ◇ change dressings   ◇ 包帯交換する
- ◇ give anesthesia   ◇ 麻酔する
- ◇ suction*   ◇ 吸引する
- ◇ insert a tube   ◇ 挿管する
- ◇ catheterize urethra   ◇ 導尿する
- ◇ give an enema   ◇ 浣腸する
- ◇ give a bed bath   ◇ 清拭する
- ◇ give first aid   ◇ 応急処置する

＊suction…動詞としても使われる

Chapter 10
Story B

In the evenings at home, I prepare a lot for the next day. I collect my patient's information, assess it and make a nursing care plan. However, implementing the plan is really difficult.

I innocently dreamed of becoming a nurse but now I'm facing that reality. Differences between what I learned at school and the actual hospital situation are greater than I thought. I wonder how long it will take me to be able to give the proper care just like the senior nurses? I still have a long way to go.

However, I have a responsibility for the patients' health even for a short period. At the hospital I met many nice people—patients who are assisting us in our nursing training in spite of their illnesses, and patients who cheered me up. They said, "Study a lot, get a lot of experience, and you'll be a very good nurse!"

I have to move forward for them, even one step at a time. Though, honestly, I can't stop my heart from wavering a little today....

Hana

Word List

- assess（2） アセスメントを行う，事前評価を行う
- nursing care plan（2） 看護計画
- implement（2） 実践する

- innocently（4） 無邪気に
- proper care（7） 適切なケア
- have a long way to go（7） 道のりは遠い，先は長い

- for a short period（8） 短期間
- cheer ~ up（10） ~を元気づける，応援する

- move forward（13） 前に進む
- one step at a time（13） 一歩ずつ
- can't stop from ~ ing（14） ~せずにはいられない
- waver（14） （心が）揺れる，迷う

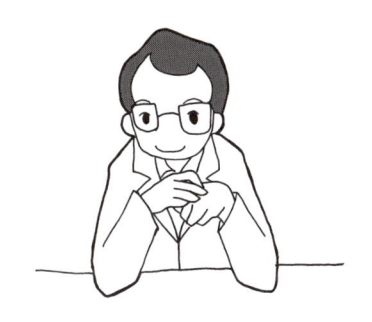

しっかり病院実習してもらいます

Chapter 10

Exercises

Ⅰ．本文の内容について選択肢の中で最もふさわしい答えを選びましょう。

1. What department do you think Hana is working in?

    (a) pediatrics　　(b) gynecology　　(c) psychiatry　　(d) orthopedics

2. What kind of personality does Hana usually have?

    (a) optimistic　　(b) pessimistic　　(c) careful　　(d) serious

3. What is Hana's feeling now?

    (a) She is moved and feeling like crying.

    (b) She is getting bored and almost giving up.

    (c) She is losing confidence but trying to move ahead.

    (d) She is getting angry but trying to be patient.

Ⅱ．ハナが研修で行ったことを本文のストーリーの順番に並べ替えましょう。ただしハナが実際には行っていないことも選択肢に混じっています。

1. Check her patient's temperature, pulse and blood pressure.
2. Distribute meals and help her patient to eat.
3. Make a nursing care plan.
4. Treat wounds by disinfecting.
5. Give a bed bath.

    (　　)→(　　)→(　　)→(　　)

Ⅲ．該当する英語を右から選びましょう。

1. 輸血　(　　)
2. 採血　(　　)
3. 麻酔　(　　)
4. 切開　(　　)
5. 注射　(　　)
6. 導尿　(　　)

(a) urethral catheterization
(b) injection
(c) incision
(d) blood sampling
(e) anesthesia
(f) blood transfusion

Speaking Tips!

● Yes それとも No?

日本語で「痛みは**あります**か？」と聞かれたとき，もし痛みがなければ「いいえ（ありません）」と答えます。しかし「痛みは**ない**ですか？」と否定文で聞かれたときは，同じく痛みがない場合でも，「はい（ありません）」と答えます。

一方英語では，"**Do** you have any pain?" と聞かれても，"**Don't** you have any pain?" と聞かれても，痛みがない場合はどちらも "**No**（I don't）" と答えます。

つまり日本語では，相手の質問が肯定文か否定文かによって「はい」「いいえ」の答え方が変わりますが，英語では，質問が肯定文か否定文かは答え方に影響しません。

医療現場での Yes / No の取り違えは大変な事態を引き起こしかねません。少しでも自信がないときは必ず "Do you mean 〜?" などと聞き返して，確認する勇気をもちましょう。

● Come それとも Go?

たとえば電話で，「今から（あなたのところに）行きます」と言うときの英語は何でしょう？「行く」は "go" だから "I'm going" でしょうか？ いえ，実際は "I'm coming" を使います。

日本語では自分を基準にして，相手に向かって「行く」のですが，英語では相手のいる位置を基準に考えて，"come"（来る）を使います。気をつけないと，これも誤解のもとですね。

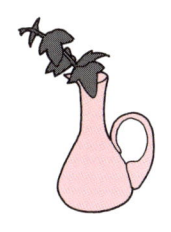

Chapter 11 A Nurse's Job

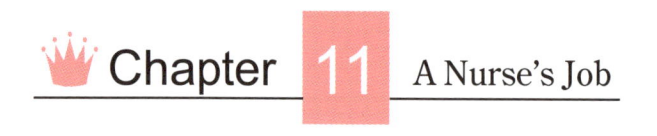

Tough, but Rewarding

Story A

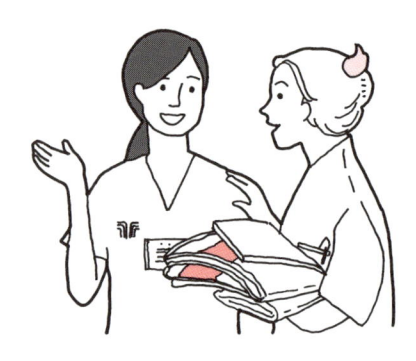

術後の患者さん，特に気をつけてあげてね
了解！

Dear Hana,

It sounds like you are having a very hard time as a student nurse. A couple of years ago, I had a chance to watch nurses working when my husband, Erik, had lung surgery for pneumothorax. I'll write about it as it may give you some idea about how nurses are working in my country.

During the surgery, Erik was totally unconscious due to the anesthesia. When he woke up in the recovery room, a nurse asked him how he was feeling. Then she checked his vital signs, IV drip and urinary catheter. She did everything very quickly and efficiently.

Later as he started feeling pain, he pushed the nurse call button. Then his bed number was shown on the small digital display boards which nurses can see everywhere in the ward. Soon the nurse came to him and he asked for a painkiller.

The next morning at 7:30 a.m., the nurse checked Erik's temperature in his ear, and explained about his medication. At 8:00 a.m., she served him breakfast and tea. The doctor came at 9:00 a.m. and instructed her to take out Erik's urinary catheter, as everything seemed fine with him. Around noon, the nurse warmed up Erik's precooked lunch in a microwave oven and brought it to him. His meal was chicken with boiled potatoes, vegetables and some bread.

Word List

tough 大変な，困難な
rewarding やりがいのある，価値のある，報われる
pneumothorax（3） 気胸*

unconscious（5） 意識がない
due to 〜（5） 〜のために
urinary catheter（7） 尿道カテーテル
quickly and efficiently（8） てきぱきと

digital display board（10） 電子掲示板
painkiller（12） 鎮痛剤

precooked（17） 調理済みの，前もって調理してある

*気胸…胸膜腔内に空気がたまること。外傷等が原因でない自然気胸は長身・やせ型の若い男性に多い病気。

Chapter 11

Dialog 16 （薬の服用）

Nurse: Here is your medicine.
Patient: When should I take it?
Nurse: Take 1 pink tablet 3 times a day after meals.
         Drink plenty of water with it.
Patient: OK.

☆ 2人1組になってDialogを練習しましょう。交代して両方の役を行います。
☆ P. 95のStep Up! Vocabularyを参考に下の会話を英語で行いましょう。
　 そのほかの単語にも入れ替えて練習しましょう。

1. A：お薬が出ていますよ。
   B：いつ飲むのですか？
   A：緑色のカプセル1錠と白い粉薬1包（packet）を
      1日2回，朝食前と夕食前に飲んでください。
      少し眠くなるかもしれません。
   B：わかりました。

2. A：お薬が出ていますよ。
   B：いつ使う（use）のですか？
   A：点眼薬は1日1回，寝る前に使ってください。
      軟膏は1日1回，風呂上がりに（after taking a bath）
      塗って（spread）ください。
   B：わかりました。

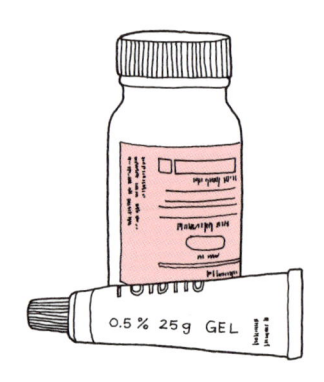

お薬はきちんと飲んでくださいね

Step Up! Vocabulary

薬の種類と服用法　Medications

- ☐ tablet, pill　　　　　　　　　　☐ 錠剤
- ☐ capsule　　　　　　　　　　　☐ カプセル
- ☐ powder　　　　　　　　　　　☐ 粉薬
- ☐ granule　　　　　　　　　　　☐ 顆粒
- ☐ syrup　　　　　　　　　　　　☐ シロップ
- ☐ inhalant　　　　　　　　　　　☐ 吸入薬
- ☐ inhaler　　　　　　　　　　　☐ 吸入器
- ☐ eye drops　　　　　　　　　　☐ 点眼薬
- ☐ suppository　　　　　　　　　☐ 座薬
- ☐ ointment　　　　　　　　　　☐ 軟膏
- ☐ cream　　　　　　　　　　　　☐ クリーム

- ☐ cold medicine　　　　　　　　☐ 風邪薬
- ☐ cough medicine　　　　　　　☐ 咳止め
- ☐ fever reducer　　　　　　　　☐ 解熱剤
- ☐ painkiller　　　　　　　　　　☐ 鎮痛剤
- ☐ sedative　　　　　　　　　　　☐ 鎮静剤
- ☐ stomach medicine　　　　　　☐ 胃薬
- ☐ laxative　　　　　　　　　　　☐ 下剤
- ☐ antibiotic　　　　　　　　　　☐ 抗生物質
- ☐ Chinese herbal medicine　　　☐ 漢方薬

- ☐ prescription drug　　　　　　　☐ 処方薬（医師の処方が必要）
- ☐ over-the-counter drug [OTC drug]　☐ 市販薬（医師の処方は不要）

- ☐ once a day　　　　　　　　　　☐ 1日1回
- ☐ twice a day, two times a day　　☐ 1日2回
- ☐ three times a day　　　　　　　☐ 1日3回
- ☐ every ~ hours　　　　　　　　☐ ~時間ごとに
- ☐ before meal(s)　　　　　　　　☐ 食前に
- ☐ after meal(s)　　　　　　　　　☐ 食後に
- ☐ between meals　　　　　　　　☐ 食間に
- ☐ before going to bed　　　　　　☐ 寝る前に
- ☐ when you have a fever　　　　☐ 熱が出た時に
- ☐ when you feel pain　　　　　　☐ 痛みがある時に

Tough, but Rewarding

薬の服用

Chapter 11
Story B

The nurse in charge of Erik looked really busy, running around to help six patients who were calling her frequently. In the afternoon, however, Erik and I enjoyed a short conversation with her, including precautions after discharge from the hospital.

While talking, I asked her if she liked her job. It looked tough and stressful being a nurse with such heavy responsibilities, always watching over people's lives and health.

She replied immediately. "I'm glad to work here. It's good to feel I can use my nursing skills to help sick people. Nurses can help patients have a more comfortable time in the hospital, and listen to any worries they may have."

"Sometimes I suffer from a lack of confidence, especially when I face difficult situations, but I've never thought about quitting. This job requires a lot of patience but I think I can keep calm even under pressure if I have enough medical knowledge and experience." Erik and I felt very grateful for her professionalism and devotion.

Hana, you have just started on the path to becoming a full-fledged nurse. Someday you will be proud of yourself as a highly-trained, trusted nurse who is always ready to help sick people. Hang in there, Hana, for your future patients and for your dream!

Lots of hugs,

Lotta

Word List

run around（1） 走り回る
precaution（3） 注意，用心すること

being a nurse（6） 看護師であること
watch over（6） 見守る，世話をする

any worries they may have（10） 患者が抱きがちな不安

from a lack of confidence（11） 自信がなくなって
face difficult situations（11） 困難な状況に直面する
quit（12） （看護の）仕事をやめる
keep calm（13） 冷静さを保つ
devotion（15） 献身（的な看護）

start on the path to becoming ～（16） ～になるための道を歩み始める
full-fledged（16） 一人前の
highly-trained（17） 高度な訓練を受けた
ready to ～（18） いつでも～できる
hang in there（18） がんばる，勇気を出す

lots of hugs（20） 愛をこめて（hug＝ぎゅっと抱きしめること）

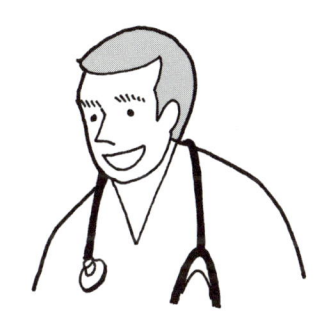

Chapter 11

Exercises

Ⅰ. 本文の内容について正しい答えを選びましょう。

1. Where did the nurse check Erik's temperature?

    (a) armpit   (b) mouth   (c) ear   (d) anus

2. What kind of anesthesia was Erik given during the surgery?

    (a) local anesthesia   (b) general anesthesia   (c) no anesthesia

3. What kind of medicine did Erik ask for after the surgery?

    (a) fever reducer   (b) sedative

    (c) laxative   (d) painkiller

4. What did the nurse NOT check about Erik in the stories?

    (a) his vital signs   (b) his incision

    (c) his urinary catheter   (d) his intravenous drip

Ⅱ. 該当する日本語を右から選びましょう。

1. tablet   (　)   (a) 座薬
2. ointment   (　)   (b) カプセル
3. granule   (　)   (c) 顆粒
4. capsule   (　)   (d) 軟膏
5. suppository (　)   (e) シロップ
6. syrup   (　)   (f) 錠剤

Ⅲ. もしあなたがハナだったら，ロッタのこのメールを読んでどんな返事を書きますか？　看護や福祉の仕事についてあなたはどんな思いをもっていますか？　簡単な英語で返事のメールを書き，これからハナがどうするか，あなた自身の考えるこのストーリーの結末を作ってみましょう。（P.101 に書きましょう）

Reading Tips!

● **医療現場でのスウェーデン・マッサージ**

スウェーデンでは約200年前にマッサージの開発研究が始まりました。人の手の温かみを通して筋肉の緊張をほぐし，ストレスを和らげるための技術が，その後長い間研究されてきました。普通科の高校でもマッサージ技術の選択授業を行うところもあって，大切な技能の1つと考えられているようです。

この国で始まったマッサージの1つに「タクティール」という，皮膚をやさしくなでるように行うものがあります。とくに認知症や緩和ケアなどの医療・福祉場面で盛んに用いられるようになり，一定の効果が報告されているそうです。筋肉を押したり揉んだりする従来のマッサージとは違い，そっとさするような穏やかなマッサージで，実際にやってもらうと気持ちがとても落ち着いて，ついうっとり…。マッサージを行う側も穏やかな気持ちになれるのが特徴で，患者とのコミュニケーション方法としても，認知症高齢者や末期患者，ADHD児などのケアに活用されています。

● **ノーベル賞の意外な一面**

毎年12月10日にストックホルムでノーベル賞の授賞式が行われます。これは最高の学者にのみ与えられる大変権威ある「お堅い」賞だと思われるかもしれませんが，その授賞式は意外にアットホーム。歌手やオーケストラが次々に演奏し，曲と曲の合間に国王から賞が授与されるので，式典というよりはまるで素敵なコンサートのようです。後方観客席からはフラッシュがおかまいなしにピカピカたかれています。

式典終了後は，客席にいた受賞者の家族や友人たちがどんどんステージに上がって来て，お互いに抱き合ったり，記念写真を撮り合ったりして受賞を喜びます。意外にカジュアルなムードで，見ているほうもなんだか微笑ましくなる光景です。

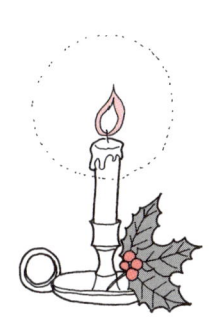

Chapter 12 Epilogue

In the Future

Dear Lotta,

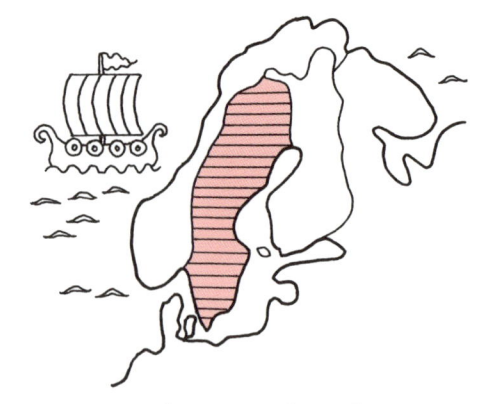

I read your e-mail and was encouraged a lot by your words. Even though my hospital training was sometimes tough, I was able to learn many things. I was so happy when my patient got better and was discharged from the hospital. I felt pain in my heart when I saw patients and their families suffering.

It won't be easy as I must study hard, but now I really want to become a nurse. I not only want to be trusted as a medical professional but also want to become a nurse who can understand patients' feelings. After getting more experience, I'm sure I'll have pride and confidence in my work.

By the way, Lotta, you may be surprised to hear this. Sometimes I'm dating Mats! I invited him to my grandpa's birthday, and then he invited me to an ice hockey game. Since then I've been seeing him sometimes. He's so cool!

Lotta, when I read your e-mails I think of you living so far away. Your country's natural environment, social systems and way of thinking are very different from Japan's. One day, I'd like to visit your hometown and see where you and Mats grew up. I'd love to meet your cute students, too.

Vacation season is coming soon. I hope you and your family have an enjoyable holiday!

Love,

Hana

In the Future

Appendix

Step Up! Vocabulary

人体外部　External Body Parts

☐ head	☐ 頭	☐ chest	☐ 胸
☐ forehead	☐ 額	☐ abdomen	☐ 腹
☐ chin	☐ あご	☐ back	☐ 背中
☐ face	☐ 顔	☐ lower back	☐ 腰
☐ eye	☐ 目	☐ buttock(s)	☐ 尻
☐ ear	☐ 耳	☐ genital(s)	☐ 性器
☐ nose	☐ 鼻	☐ penis	☐ 陰茎
☐ nostril	☐ 鼻孔	☐ testicle(s)	☐ 睾丸
☐ mouth	☐ 口	☐ anus	☐ 肛門
☐ lip	☐ 唇		
		☐ leg	☐ 脚
☐ neck	☐ 首	☐ thigh	☐ 太もも
☐ shoulder	☐ 肩	☐ knee	☐ 膝
☐ arm	☐ 腕	☐ shin	☐ すね
☐ armpit	☐ わきの下	☐ calf	☐ ふくらはぎ
☐ elbow	☐ ひじ	☐ ankle	☐ 足首
☐ wrist	☐ 手首	☐ foot	☐ 足
☐ hand	☐ 手	☐ heel	☐ かかと
☐ finger	☐ 指	☐ toe	☐ 足の指
☐ thumb	☐ 親指	☐ sole	☐ 足の裏
☐ nail	☐ 爪		

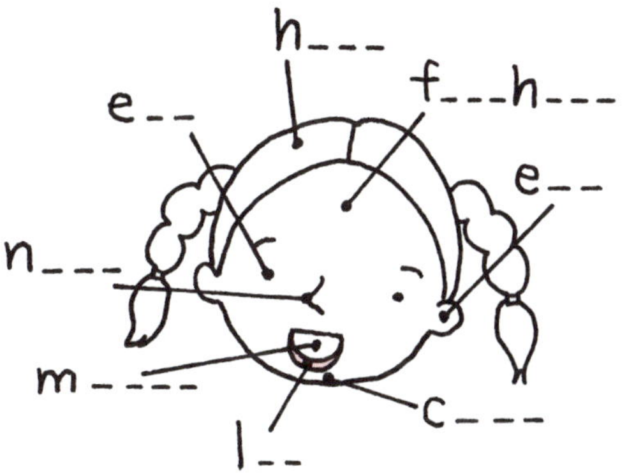
h___
f___h___
e__
e__
n___
m____
l__
c___

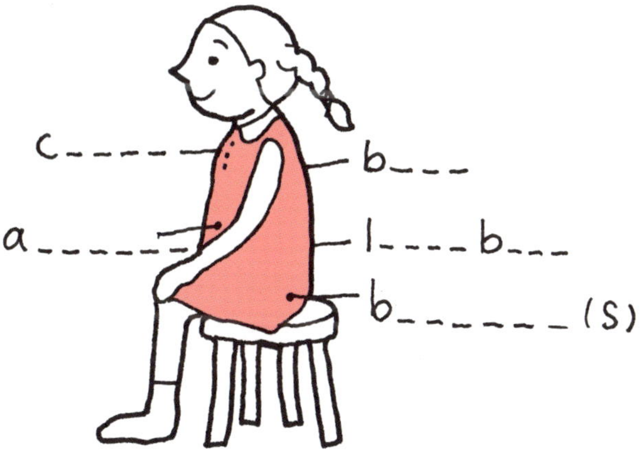
c_____
b___
a______
l___b___
b_______(s)

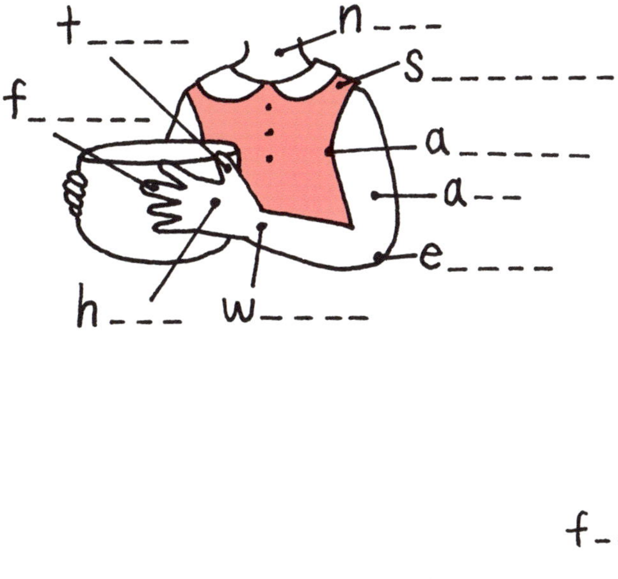
t____
n___
s_______
f_____
a______
a__
e____
h___
w____

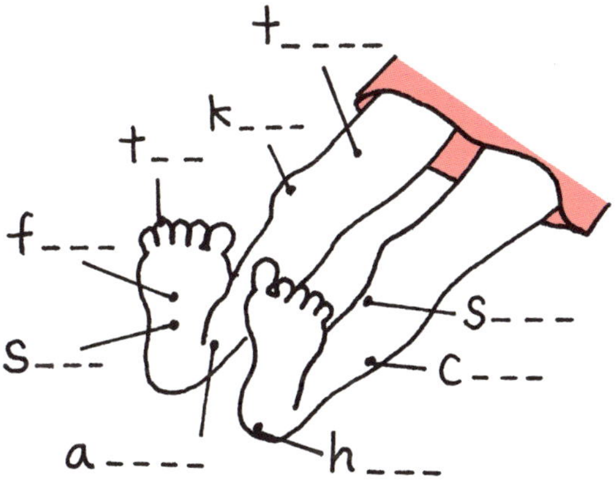
t____
k___
t__
f___
s___
s___
c___
a____
h___

Appendix

人体内部　Internal Body Parts

☐ brain	☐ 脳	☐ gallbladder	☐ 胆嚢 (たんのう)
☐ eardrum	☐ 鼓膜	☐ spleen	☐ 脾臓 (ひぞう)
☐ throat	☐ 喉	☐ kidney	☐ 腎臓 (じんぞう)
☐ tonsil(s)	☐ 扁桃腺	☐ pancreas	☐ 膵臓 (すいぞう)
☐ tooth / teeth（複数）	☐ 歯	☐ bladder	☐ 膀胱 (ぼうこう)
☐ tongue	☐ 舌	☐ urethra	☐ 尿道
☐ esophagus	☐ 食道	☐ ovary	☐ 卵巣
☐ stomach	☐ 胃	☐ uterus	☐ 子宮
☐ small intestine(s)	☐ 小腸	☐ vagina	☐ 膣
☐ duodenum	☐ 十二指腸		
☐ large intestine	☐ 大腸	☐ blood vessel	☐ 血管
☐ colon	☐ 結腸	☐ artery	☐ 動脈
☐ rectum	☐ 直腸	☐ vein	☐ 静脈
☐ appendix	☐ 虫垂		
		☐ muscle	☐ 筋肉
☐ lung	☐ 肺	☐ bone	☐ 骨
☐ heart	☐ 心臓	☐ spine	☐ 脊椎
☐ liver	☐ 肝臓	☐ rib	☐ 肋骨

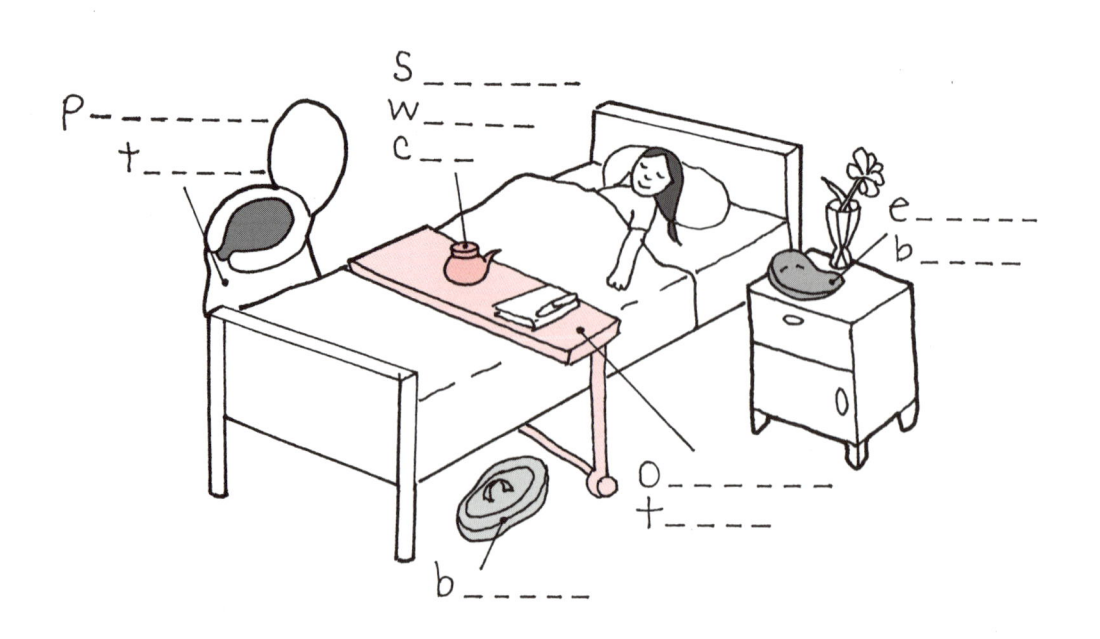

p _ _ _ _ _ _
t _ _ _ _
s _ _ _ _ _ _
w _ _ _ _ _
c _ _ _
e _ _ _ _ _
b _
o _
t _ _ _ _
b _ _ _ _ _

院内の備品　Hospital Equipment

- ☐ stethoscope
- ☐ thermometer
- ☐ blood pressure gauge
- ☐ vital signs monitor
- ☐ syringe
- ☐ tourniquet
- ☐ forceps
- ☐ penlight

- ☐ latex glove(s)
- ☐ surgical mask
- ☐ bandage
- ☐ cotton ball
- ☐ gauze

- ☐ examination table
- ☐ stretcher
- ☐ bedside table
- ☐ overbed table
- ☐ side rail
- ☐ pillow
- ☐ pillowcase
- ☐ sheet
- ☐ blanket

- ☐ spouted water cup
- ☐ emesis〔kidney〕basin
- ☐ portable toilet
- ☐ bedpan
- ☐ urine bottle
- ☐ diaper

- ☐ 聴診器
- ☐ 体温計
- ☐ 血圧計
- ☐ バイタルサインモニター
- ☐ 注射器
- ☐ 駆血帯（くけつたい）
- ☐ 鉗子（かんし）
- ☐ ペンライト

- ☐ ゴム手袋
- ☐ マスク
- ☐ 包帯
- ☐ 脱脂綿
- ☐ ガーゼ

- ☐ 診察台
- ☐ ストレッチャー，担架
- ☐ 床頭台（しょうとうだい）
- ☐ オーバーテーブル
- ☐ ベッドの柵
- ☐ 枕
- ☐ 枕カバー
- ☐ シーツ
- ☐ 毛布

- ☐ 吸いのみ
- ☐ 膿盆
- ☐ ポータブルトイレ
- ☐ ベッドパン，おまる
- ☐ しびん
- ☐ おむつ

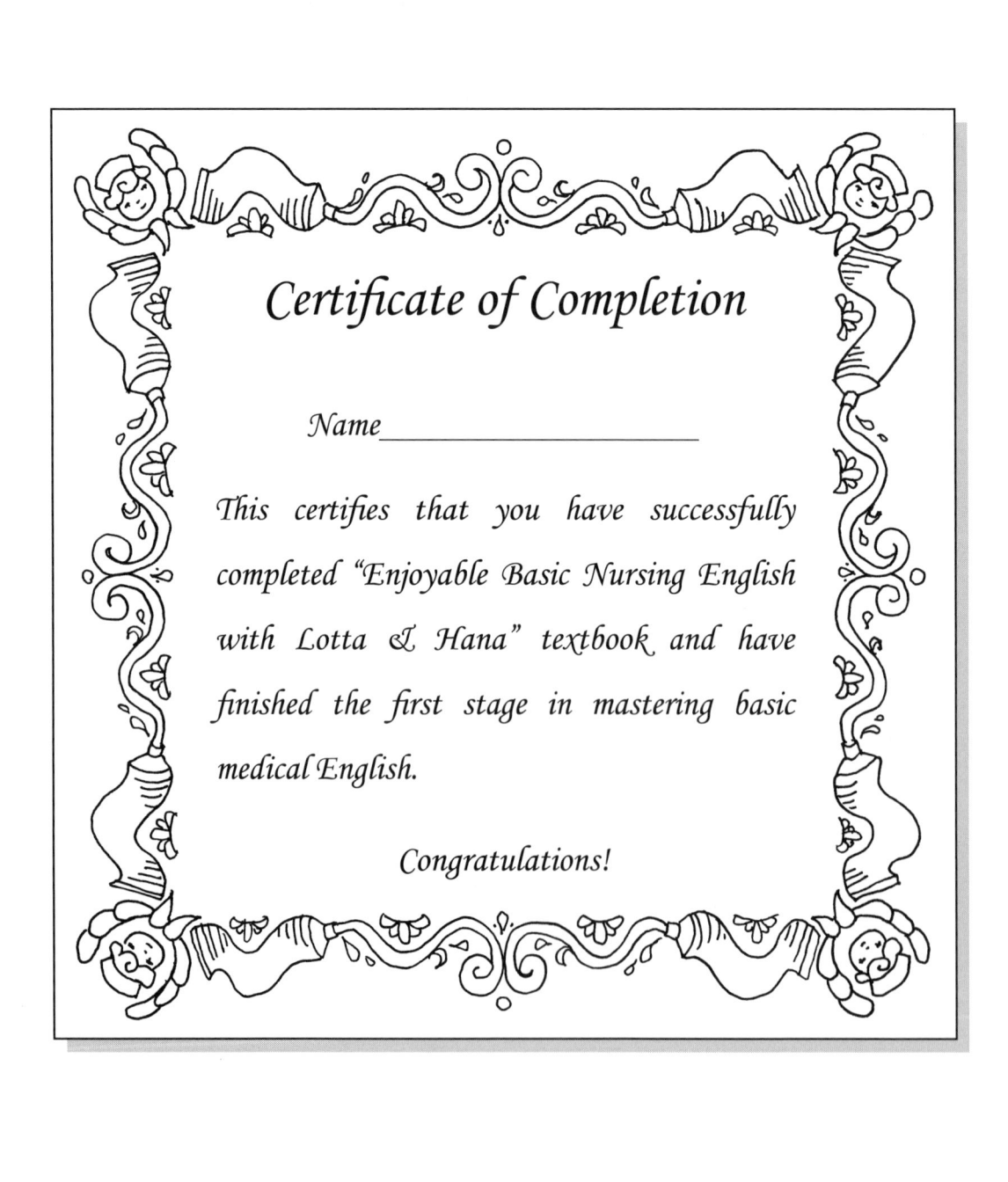

Certificate of Completion

*Name*_____

This certifies that you have successfully completed "Enjoyable Basic Nursing English with Lotta & Hana" textbook and have finished the first stage in mastering basic medical English.

Congratulations!

Glossary

＊訳語は原則として本書で使われる意味だけを示した。

A

abdominal　腹部の　18, 40, 44
abdominal circumference　腹囲　44
actual　実際の　84
advanced　進んだ　6
AIDS　エイズ　81
aim　目的，目指す　60, 74
allergy　アレルギー　11
allow　許可する，認める　33
alone　〜だけの　41
Alzheimer's disease　アルツハイマー病　80
amount　量　66
anemia　貧血　38
anesthesia　麻酔　33
annual　年に一度の　74
antibiotic　抗生物質　95
apparent　明らかな，はっきり見える　77
appendicitis　虫垂炎　80
appetite　食欲　59
appetite loss　食欲不振　59
appointment　予約　20, 26
appointment card　予約カード　26
appropriate　適切な　77
assess　アセスメントを行う，事前評価を行う　88
assign　割り当てる　38
assist　助ける　56
assistance　支援　56, 60, 69
assistance dog　介助犬　69
asthma　喘息　80
attach　添付する　33, 60
attend　出席する　38
authority　当局　66
average　平均(の)　33

B

backache　背部痛，腰痛　18
barley　大麦　55
barrier-free　バリアフリー(の)　70
basically　基本的に　20
basis　基礎　15
bed bath　清拭　84
beforehand　前もって　84
belly　腹部　41

blood　血　38, 44, 84, 87
blood pressure　血圧　44, 84
blood sampling　採血　87
blood test　血液検査　38
blood transfusion　輸血　87
bloody stool　血便　59
bloody urine　血尿　59
body mass index　肥満度指数，体格指数　44
bonito　カツオ　55
bowel movement　排便，便通　59
breast milk　母乳　33
breathe　呼吸する　30
breathing technique　呼吸法　30
bronchial　気管支の　80
bronchitis　気管支炎　80
burp　ゲップ(する)　59

C

Caesarian section　帝王切開　38
caloric restriction　カロリー制限　59
cancer　悪性腫瘍，がん　81
cane　杖　68, 69
capsule　カプセル　95
cardiology (department of)　循環器内科　48
carefully　注意深く　15, 74
cashier　会計(係)　23, 26
cataract　白内障　81
catheterize　カテーテルを入れる　87
celebrate　祝う　48
cerebral　(大)脳の　80
cerebral hemorrhage　脳出血　80
cerebral infarction　脳梗塞　80
checkup　健診　38
chest　胸　18
chickenpox　水ぼうそう　81
childbirth　出産　41
chill　悪寒　18
chopstick(s)　はし　36
chronic　慢性の　56
circumstance　状況　52
cirrhosis　肝硬変　80
classify　等級に分ける　66
clinic　診療所，クリニック　20, 23
clinical psychologist　臨床心理士　51
collect　収集する　88

colonoscopy　大腸(内視)鏡検査　44
comfortable　快適な　52, 84, 96
complete　完了する，完成させる　20
computerized tomography [CT scan]　CT 検査，コンピュータ断層撮影　44
concern　心配事　58
confidence　自信　96, 100
congratulations　おめでとう　38
constipation　便秘　59
contract　契約　66
contraction(s)　陣痛，(子宮の)収縮　30
convenient　都合のよい，便利な　20
cool　素敵な，かっこいい　100
cooperate　協力する　23
cough　咳　18
cramp(s)　けいれん　18
crutch(es)　松葉杖　69
custard　カスタード(卵・砂糖などを煮たり蒸したりした食品)　55

D

daily　毎日　56
dawn　夜明け　33
delivery　分娩，出産　30, 33, 41
delivery room　分娩室　33
dementia　認知症　56, 80
depression　うつ病　81
detail　詳細　15
develop　発展させる，発展する　48
development　開発，発展　52
device　工夫，装置　70
devil's tongue　こんにゃく　55
devotion　献身　96
diabetes (mellitus)　糖尿病　81
diagnosis　診断　15
diarrhea　下痢　59
dietitian　栄養士　51
diphtheria　ジフテリア　81
disability　障がい　8, 52, 66, 70, 73, 74, 77
disabled　障がいのある　70
discharge (from hospital)　退院(させる)　33, 96, 100
disinfect　消毒する　84

107

Glossary

disinfection 消毒 87
distribute 配る 84
dizziness めまい 18
dressing 包帯，手当て用品（ガーゼ，軟膏など） 84
dressing change 包帯交換 87
duodenal ulcer 十二指腸潰瘍 80

E

earache 耳痛 12
echogram 超音波検査 40, 44
echography 超音波検査 44
efficiently 能率的に 92
elderly 年配の人，高齢者 48
electrocardiogram［ECG, EKG］ 心電図（検査） 44
electroencephalogram［EEG］ 脳波（検査） 44
electronic prescription system 電子処方システム 15
embarrassing 恥ずかしい 84
emergency alarm 非常ベル，緊急ボタン 48
emergency exit 非常口 36
emergency room［ER］ 救急処置室 26
employ 雇う 66
encourage 勇気づける，奨励する 60, 70, 74, 100
enema 浣腸 87
energetic 元気な 33
enjoyable 楽しい 100
ENT (Ear, Nose and Throat) 耳鼻咽喉科 12
environment 環境 60
epilepsy てんかん 80
examine 診察する 15
exchange 交換，交流（する） 6, 8, 60

F

face 直面する 88
family history 家族歴 11
favorite お気に入りの，大好きな 52, 56, 60
ferment 発酵させる 55
fever 熱 17, 95
fever reducer 解熱剤 95
financial 財政的な 52
first visit 初診 20
fist 握りこぶし 86
flake 薄片，フレーク 55
four-person room ４人部屋 33

fracture 骨折 81
freedom 自由 66
frequent urination 頻尿 59
frequently 頻繁に 96
full-fledged 一人前の 96
fundamental 基本的な 60

G

gallstone(s) 胆石 80
gastric ulcer 胃潰瘍 80
gastroenteritis 胃腸炎 80
gastroscopy 胃（内視）鏡検査 44
general hospital 総合病院 15
general information 総合案内 26
general practitioner 総合医，一般医 12
generation 世代 30
go well うまくいく 38
gout 痛風 81
government 政府 41
gradually 次第に 70
granule 顆粒 95
grate （おろし金で）おろす 55
growth 成長，発育 38
gynecology 婦人科 51

H

handrail てすり 69
headache 頭痛 18
health insurance card 健康保険証 20, 22
hearing 聴力 12, 44, 69, 74
hearing aid 補聴器 69
hearing test 聴力検査 44
heart attack 心臓発作 80
heart rate 心拍数 44
heartbeat 心臓の鼓動，心拍 38
height 身長 11, 41
hepatitis A［B］［C］ A［B］［C］型肝炎 80
hiccup(s) しゃっくり 18
high-level 高度な 56
highly-trained 高度な訓練を受けた 96
hire 雇う 66
hives じんましん 81
home care 在宅介護 56, 66
home care provider 在宅介護事業者 66
home care worker 訪問介護員，ホームヘルパー 56
homelike わが家のような，家庭的な 60

hometown 故郷 100
honestly 正直に 84, 88
hospital shop （病院の）売店 36
hospitalize 入院させる 41
housework 家事 66
housing 住居，住宅 48, 56, 60
hypertension 高血圧 80

I

ice hockey アイスホッケー 100
immediately すぐに，直ちに 41, 96
improve 改善する 23, 60
incision 切開 87
include 含む 66
income 収入 60
increase 増す 70
independently 独立して，自由に，自主的に 66
individual 個人の 60, 77
influenza［flu］ インフルエンザ 81
informed consent インフォームドコンセント（説明と同意） 15
inhalant 吸入薬 95
inhaler 吸入器 95
injection 注射 86, 87
inpatient 入院患者 30, 36
inpatient ward 入院病棟 30, 36
insert 挿入する 87
instruct 指示する 92
intensive care unit［ICU］ 集中治療室 36
internal medicine 内科 50, 51
intravenous drip［IV］ 点滴 87, 92
intubation 挿管 87
iron pill 鉄剤 38
itch かゆみ 18

J

Japanese-speaking 日本語を話す 77
jelly-like ゼリーのような 55
joint 関節 18

K

kidney failure 腎不全 80
kidney stone(s) 腎結石 80

Glossary

L

labor pain　陣痛　30
labor room　陣痛室　30
laboratory [lab] technician　検査技師　51
laxative　下剤　95
leukemia　白血病　81
life expectancy　寿命　52
life span　寿命　52
locate　位置する　74
look forward to　〜を楽しみにする　33
lump　しこり　18
lung　肺　92

M

magnetic resonance imaging [MRI]　MRI検査, 磁気共鳴断層撮影　44
massage　マッサージする　30
maternity　妊娠, 妊婦の　38
measles　麻疹　81
medical　医療の　6, 12, 15, 20, 23, 26, 33, 38, 41, 51, 56, 60, 96, 100
medical care　医療, 医療的ケア　56
medical chart　カルテ　26
medical consultation　診察　15
medical facility　医療施設　20
medical fee　医療費　38
medical questionnaire　問診票　20
medical social worker　医療ソーシャルワーカー　51
medical staff　医療スタッフ　41
medical system　医療制度　12, 15, 23
medical test　(医学)検査　23
medication　薬, 投薬　23
medication record book　お薬手帳　23
medicine　薬　15
meningitis　髄膜炎　74, 76
microwave oven　電子レンジ　92
midwife　助産師　33, 38, 41, 51
mumps　おたふく風邪　81
muscular　筋肉の　18
myocardial infarction　心筋梗塞　80

N

naked　裸の　41
nameless　名前がない　41
nation　国, 国家　8
nationality　国籍　11
native　母国の　77
natural birth　自然分娩　38
nausea　吐き気　18
needs　ニーズ, 必要性　77
neighborhood　近所　8
nephew　甥　38
newborn　新生児　33, 41
northern　北の　74
numbness　しびれ　18
nurses' station　看護師詰め所　35, 36

O

occupation　職業　11
occupational therapist [OT]　作業療法士　51
occur　起こる　60
ointment　軟膏　95
operating room　手術室　36
orthopedics　整形外科　51
oto (rhino) laryngology　耳鼻(咽喉)科　51
outpatient　外来患者　12, 20, 26
outpatient ward　外来病棟　12, 20, 26

P

painful　痛い　33
painkiller　鎮痛剤　92, 95
painting　絵画　15
palpitation(s)　動悸　18
pancreatitis　膵炎　80
paste　ペースト, 練り製品　55
path　道　96
patient　患者　15, 20, 23, 84, 88, 96
patient ID card　診察券　20
patient registration form　診療申込書　20
payment　支払い　66
peaceful　至福の, 穏やかな　41
pediatrics　小児科　15, 51
pharmacist　薬剤師　51
pharmacy　薬局　15, 26
physical　身体的な　51, 52, 66, 77
physical care　身体介護　66
physical therapist [PT]　理学療法士　51
pickled　酢漬けにした　55
pill　錠剤　38, 95
play area　遊び場　15
plenty　たくさん　94
plum　ウメ, プラム　55
pneumonia　肺炎　80
pneumothorax　気胸　92
polio　ポリオ, 小児まひ　81
pop music　ポップミュージック　6
potential　潜在能力, 可能性　74
powder　粉薬　95
pregnancy　妊娠　38
pregnant　妊娠した　38
prescribe　処方する　15
prescription　処方(せん)　15, 23, 26, 95
prescription fee　処方せん発行料, 投薬料　23
previous　以前の　60
previously　以前に　23, 70
pride　誇り, プライド　100
private room　個室　36
professionalism　プロ意識　96
progress　経過, 進行　30
proud　誇りにしている　60
provide　提供する　60
psychiatry　精神科　51
pulse　脈拍　44

Q

quit　辞める　96

R

range　〜(の範囲)に及ぶ　74
rash　発疹　18
reality　現実　60, 70, 88
receipt　領収書　26
receive　受け入れる　52, 66, 77
recently　最近　23
recommend　推薦する　15
recovery room　回復室　33, 36, 92
referral letter　紹介状　12
registration　登録　20
regular　定期的な　38
rehabilitation　機能回復訓練, リハビリ　48
relative　親族, 身内　56
rental charge　貸し出し料　32
require　必要とする　96
resident　住人　48
respect　尊重する　60
respiration　呼吸　44
responsibility　責任　60, 96
return visit　再診　26
rice cake　餅　55
right　権利　77

Glossary

risk　危険，リスク　60
rubella　風疹，はしか　81
runny nose　鼻水　18

S

safely　無事に，安全に　30
sales tax　消費税　60
satisfied　満足した　52, 60
sedative　鎮静剤　95
self-supporting　自立している　56
seriously ill patient　重症患者　23
serve　（飲食物を）出す　92
shape　状態，調子，体調　52
share　共有する，分け合う　6, 56, 60
shortly　まもなく　15
shortness of breath　息切れ　18
shot　注射　87
sign language　手話　69
sinusitis　副鼻腔炎　81
situation　状況，状態　12, 88, 96
sleeping pill　睡眠薬　59
sleeplessness　不眠　59
slide　すべり台　15
slight　ちょっとした　12
sneeze　くしゃみ　18
social welfare system　社会福祉制度　6, 60
sore throat　咽喉痛　18
soybean　大豆　55
soybean curd　豆腐　55
specialist　専門家　12
speech therapist [ST]　言語療法士　51
spinach　ホウレンソウ　55
sprain　ねんざ　81
sputum　痰　18
staff member　職員　48
stay　①滞在する，②～のままでいる　52, 56
stethoscope　聴診器　84
stew　煮込む　55
stitch　縫合（する）　87
stitch removal　抜糸　87
stomach medicine　胃薬　95
stomachache　胃痛　18
stool　①腰掛，スツール，②大便　25, 44, 59
stool test　検便　44
stroke　（脳）卒中　80
suction　吸引（する）　87
suffer　苦しむ，悩む　96
suppository　座薬　95
surgery　外科，手術　51, 92
surround　囲む　74
swelling　腫れ　18
symptom　兆候　17
syrup　シロップ　95

T

tablet　錠剤　95
talent　才能　70
tax　税金　60
temperature　体温　11, 84, 92
tetanus　破傷風　81
throw up　嘔吐する　59
toiletry (-ies)　洗面用具　36
tonsillitis　扁桃炎　81
toothache　歯痛　18
totally　まったく，完全に　92
traffic accident　交通事故　66, 84
treatment　治療　15, 20, 30
treatment room　処置室　30
tuberculosis　結核　81

U

ultrasound test　超音波検査　38
umbilical cord　へその緒　33
uncomfortable　不快な　84
underwear　下着　36
unexpectedly　思いがけず　84
universal design　ユニバーサルデザイン　70
unusual　珍しい　60
urethra　尿道　87
urethral catheterization　導尿　87
urinary catheter　尿道カテーテル　92
urinate　排尿する　59
urination　排尿　59
urine　尿　59
urine test　尿検査　44
user　使用者　77
uterine　子宮の　38

V

varied　さまざまな　60
vary　変わる　66
vegetarian　菜食主義者，ベジタリアン　59
vision test　視力検査　44
visiting nurse　訪問看護師　56, 58
vital signs　バイタルサイン　44, 92
vomit　嘔吐（する）　59

W

waiting room　待合室　15
walking race　競歩　74
ward　病棟　12, 20, 26, 36
weigh　～の重さがある　10, 33, 41
weight　体重　11, 41
welfare　幸福，福祉　6, 52, 60
wheelchair　車いす　66, 69, 70
wheelchair ramp　車いす用スロープ　69
wheeze　喘鳴（ぜんめい）　18
wooden　木製の　15
workplace　職場　84
wound　傷　84

X

X-ray　放射線　26, 44, 51
X-ray technician　放射線技師　51

（解答部分は必要に応じてミシン目から切り取ってご使用ください）

Sample Answers for Dialogs

Dialog 3 (Chapter 2)

1. A : What's the matter?
   B : I have a bad toothache.
   A : When did it start?
   B : It started three days ago.

2. A : What's the matter?
   B : I have a bad chest pain.
   A : When did it start?
   B : It started last night.

Dialog 4 (Chapter 2)

1. A : Do you have any other symptoms?
   B : I have a cough, too.
   A : OK, the doctor will see you shortly.

2. A : Do you have any other symptoms?
   B : I have a runny nose, too.
   A : OK, the doctor will see you shortly.

Dialog 5 (Chapter 3)

1. A : I'd like to see a doctor.
   B : Do you have your appointment card?
   A : Yes, here it is.
   B : Please put it on the counter.

2. A : I'd like to see a doctor.
   B : Do you have your patient ID card?
   A : No, this is my first visit.
   B : Please fill out this form.

Dialog 6 (Chapter 3)

1. A : Ms./Mr. ____, please enter treatment room two.
   B : Sure.
   A : Please roll up your sleeve.
   B : OK.

2. A : Ms./Mr. ____, please enter the CT room.
   B : Sure.
   A : Please lie face up on the bed.
   B : OK.

Dialog 7 (Chapter 4)

1. A : What should I bring when I enter the hospital?
   B : Please bring chopsticks and a cup.
   A : Can I buy a cup at the hospital shop?
   B : Yes.

2. A : What should I bring when I enter the hospital?
   B : Please bring slippers and a bath towel.
   A : Can I rent a bath towel?
   B : No, but you can buy one at the hospital shop.

Dialog 8 (Chapter 4)

1. A : Excuse me, where is the dining room?
   B : It's across from the lobby.
   A : When is it open?
   B : It is open from 11 a.m. to 8 p.m.

2. A : Excuse me, where is the shower room?
   B : It's to the right of the bathroom.
   A : When is it open?
   B : It is open from 2 to 6:30 p.m.

Dialog 9 (Chapter 5)

1. A : You are going to have a brain MRI today.
   B : What kind of test is that?
   A : It's to check your brain using magnetic waves.

2. A : You are going to have an electrocardiogram (ECG, EKG) today.
   B : What kind of test is that?
   A : It's to check your heart using weak electric signals.

Sample Answers for Dialogs

Dialog 10 (Chapter 5)

1. A : How high is your blood pressure now?
   B : It's 150 over 90 (one fifty over ninety).
   A : It's a little high.

2. A : How tall is your child now?
   B : He/She is 90 cm (tall).
   A : He/She is really big now!

Dialog 11 (Chapter 6)

1. A : Which department are you going to today?
   B : I'm going to cardiology.
   A : Please go straight and turn left at the second corner.
   B : Thank you.

2. A : Which department are you going to today?
   B : I'm going to orthopedics.
   A : Please go to the second floor.
   B : Thank you.

Dialog 12 (Chapter 7)

1. A : Do you have any health concerns?
   B : I have to go to the toilet many times.
   A : How many times did you urinate today?
   B : 10 times.

2. A : Do you have any health concerns?
   B : I have no appetite.
   A : How many times did you have bowel movements yesterday?
   B : None.

Dialog 13 (Chapter 8)

1. A : Can you dress by yourself?
   B : Yes, I can.
   A : Can you go up stairs by yourself?
   B : Yes, but I need handrails.

2. A : Can you walk by yourself?
   B : No, I need a wheelchair.
   A : Can you take a bath by yourself?
   B : No, I need help.

Dialog 14 (Chapter 9)

1. A : Have you ever had a serious disease?
   B : I had pneumonia two years ago.
   A : Do you have any problems now?
   B : No, I'm fine now.

2. A : Have you ever had a serious disease?
   B : I had leukemia when I was 47 years old.
   A : Do you have any problems now?
   B : Yes, I'm still receiving treatment.

Dialog 15 (Chapter 10)

1. I'll give you an IV.
   Please don't move.

2. I'll give you an enema.
   Please hold it in as long as possible.

3. I'll disinfect your wound.
   It might sting a little.

4. The doctor will insert a tube through your nose.
   Please relax.

Dialog 16 (Chapter 11)

1. A : Here is your medicine.
   B : When should I take it?
   A : Take 1 green capsule and 1 packet of white powder twice a day, before breakfast and dinner. You might feel a little sleepy.
   B : OK.

2. A : Here is your medicine.
   B : When should I use it?
   A : Use the eye drops once a day before going to bed. Spread the ointment once a day after taking a bath.
   B : OK.

Answers for Exercises

Chapter 2
Ⅰ. 1. b   2. c   3. d

Ⅱ. (2) → (5) → (6) → (4) → (1) → (3)

Ⅲ. 1. f   2. d   3. h   4. c   5. a   6. b
   7. e   8. g

Chapter 3
Ⅰ. 1. c   2. a   3. b

Ⅱ. (4) → (2) → (3) → (1)

Ⅲ. 1. d   2. e   3. b   4. f   5. c   6. a

Chapter 4
Ⅰ. 1. ×   2. ×   3. ×   4. ○   5. ○

Ⅱ. (6) → (2) → (1) → (3) → (5)

Ⅲ. 1. He was really moved when the baby was born.
   2. Mari gave her baby breast milk for the first time.

Ⅳ. 1. e   2. f   3. d   4. b   5. a   6. c

Chapter 5
Ⅰ. 1. ○   2. ×   3. ×   4. ○   5. ×   6. ×

Ⅱ. 1. one hundred (and) fifty-eight centimeters
   2. forty-six point three kilograms
   3. thirty-seven point five degrees (Celsius/centigrade)
   4. one thirty-five over eighty-two

Ⅲ. 1. c   2. e   3. f   4. b   5. d   6. a

Chapter 6
Ⅰ. 1. c   2. a   3. d

Ⅱ. 1. (The number) of older parents living with children is decreasing.
   2. Grandpa goes to a local senior day care center (regularly).

Ⅲ. 1. c   2. e   3. f   4. b   5. a   6. d

Speaking Tips!
1. B   2. A   3. O   4. D   5. G   6. N
7. H   8. I   9. K   10. L   11. F   12. C
13. M   14. J   15. E

Chapter 7
Ⅰ. 1. c   2. c   3. b

Ⅱ. 1. b   2. c   3. a

Ⅲ. 1. d   2. f   3. e   4. b   5. a   6. c

Chapter 8
Ⅰ. 1. ×   2. ○   3. ×   4. ○   5. ×

Ⅱ. 1. Awareness about a barrier-free society is increasing (in Japan).
   2. She attended a Japanese festival supported by volunteers.

Ⅲ. 1. c   2. a   3. e   4. f   5. d   6. b

Chapter 9
Ⅰ. 1. ×   2. ○   3. ○   4. ×   5. ○

Ⅱ. 1. Fifty children have minor to more serious disabilities.
   2. Children with allergies are given specially cooked lunches.

Ⅲ. 1. c   2. d   3. e   4. f   5. g   6. i
   7. h   8. j   9. a   10. b

Answers

Chapter 10

Ⅰ. 1. d　2. a　3. c

Ⅱ. (2) → (1) → (5) → (3)

Ⅲ. 1. f　2. d　3. e　4. c　5. b　6. a

Chapter 11

Ⅰ. 1. c　2. b　3. d　4. b

Ⅱ. 1. f　2. d　3. c　4. b　5. a　6. e

Answers for Word Searches / Crossword Puzzles

Word Search 1 　(P. 28)

A	Q	U	C	H	I	L	L	J	M	W	D
O	N	P	N	V	T	X	Q	N	A	B	I
V	K	H	A	P	P	Y	U	P	T	Y	P
F	E	V	E	R	E	M	J	L	A	M	I
P	Z	I	J	E	B	E	C	M	H	Z	N
F	E	L	U	N	W	L	P	S	G	H	E
C	E	B	E	P	E	P	A	G	U	I	B
G	N	S	T	C	N	R	Q	P	O	N	S
O	S	T	O	M	A	C	H	A	C	H	E
W	A	U	X	H	O	L	I	D	A	Y	S
Z	O	T	F	R	M	U	T	U	P	S	Y
E	H	C	A	D	A	E	H	O	V	E	R

1. 頭痛　2. 胃痛, 腹痛　3. 熱　4. 悪寒　5. 咳
6. くしゃみ　7. 痰　8. 発疹

Word Search 2 　(P. 64)

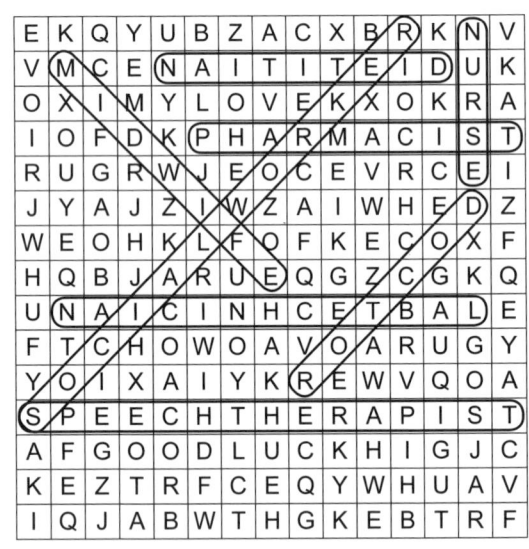

E	K	Q	Y	U	B	Z	A	C	X	B	R	K	N	V
V	M	C	E	N	A	I	T	I	T	E	I	D	U	K
O	X	I	M	Y	L	O	V	E	K	X	O	K	R	A
I	O	F	D	K	P	H	A	R	M	A	C	I	S	T
R	U	G	R	W	J	E	O	C	E	V	R	C	E	I
J	Y	A	J	Z	I	W	Z	A	I	W	H	E	D	Z
W	E	O	H	K	L	X	F	O	F	K	E	C	O	X
H	Q	B	J	A	R	U	E	Q	G	Z	C	G	K	Q
U	N	A	I	C	I	N	H	C	E	T	B	A	L	E
F	T	C	H	O	W	O	A	V	O	A	R	U	G	Y
Y	O	I	X	A	I	Y	K	R	E	W	V	Q	O	A
S	P	E	E	C	H	T	H	E	R	A	P	I	S	T
A	F	G	O	O	D	L	U	C	K	H	I	G	J	C
K	E	Z	T	R	F	C	E	Q	Y	W	H	U	A	V
I	Q	J	A	B	W	T	H	G	K	E	B	T	R	F

1. 看護師　2. 助産師　3. 医師　4. 検査技師
5. 栄養士　6. 薬剤師　7. 言語療法士　8. ソーシャルワーカー, 社会福祉士

Crossword Puzzle 1 　(P. 46)

ACROSS
6. NURSES' STATION　（看護師詰め所）
7. RECOVERY ROOM　（回復室）
8. OUTPATIENT WARD　（外来病棟）

DOWN
1. RECEPTION　（受付）
2. CASHIER　（会計）
3. PHARMACY　（薬局）
4. WAITING ROOM　（待合室）
5. INPATIENT WARD　（入院病棟）

Crossword Puzzle 2 　(P. 82)

ACROSS
2. NEUROLOGY　（神経内科）
6. PSYCHIATRY　（精神科）
7. SURGERY　（外科）
8. DENTISTRY　（歯科）

DOWN
1. PEDIATRICS　（小児科）
3. RADIOLOGY　（放射線科）
4. OBSTETRICS　（産科）
5. UROLOGY　（泌尿器科）